Understanding Antiviral Immunity:
Lessons from COVID-19 patient responses

Gnatoulma Katawa

Publisher: Upway Books
Authors: Gnatoulma Katawa
Title: Understanding Antiviral Immunity: Lessons from COVID-19 patient responses
ISBN: 978-1-917916-63-9
Cover Designed on Canva: www.canva.com

contact@upwaybooks.com
www.upwaybooks.com

Contents

Chapiter 1: Human Coronaviruses

INTRODUCTION

Humanity has been struggling against pathogens. Theses pathogens cause parasitic diseases[1], bacterial infectionsand viral such us HIV[2], hepatitis B[3, 4] and recent Covid-19 causes by SARS-CoV-2[5].*Coronaviridae* are single-stranded, positive-sense RNA viruses enveloped non-segmented, designatedafter their corona- or crown-like on electron microscopy[6, 7]. The International Committee on Taxonomy of Viruses (ICTV) established in 1975 the family of *Coronavirus*, which was divided into two genera in April 1992: the *coronavirusgenus* and the *torovirusgenus*[8]. Three genetically and serogically groups of *coronavirus genus* have been described [9]. Group I compriseHuman CoV-229E (HCoV-229E), Human CoV-NL63 (HCoV-NL63) and Feline infectious peritonitis virus (FIPV).GroupIIincludesHuman CoV-OC43 (HCoV-OC43), Human CoV-HKU1 (HCoV-KHU1), Severe acute respiratory syndrome-CoV(SARS-CoV) and Mouse hepatitis virus (MHV). The group III contains bronchitis Infectious virus (IBV)[9-11] . The viral taxonomy has been regularly reviewed according to the following orders: the order of *Nidovirales*, created in 1996, which currently groups together three families (*Coronaviridae*, *Arteriviridae* and *Roniviridae*). These viruses have in common the organization of the RNA genome and the replication strategy but differ in their morphology, their capsid structure and the size of their genome which ranges from 13 000 nucleotides for *arterivirus* to 31 000 nucleotides for *coronavirus* [12]. Thus, group I and II coronaviruses infect mammals, including humans and group III coronaviruess are a group of avian viruses[13].

The classification of SARS-CoV has been much debated and the various phylogenetic analyzes proposed either to place it in a fourth group, or in a group II "extended". Finally, the latter solution was adopted and currently subdivided group II into 2a and 2b, and includes SARS-CoV as well as all the "SARS-CoV-like" or SL-CoV virus described in the different animal species[14, 15] . In the 1960s, Human CoV (HCoV) comprisedsix strains: 229E, OC43 are most known than B814, OC16, OC37 and OC48. In 2003, the Chinese population was infected with a virus causing severe acute respiratory syndrome (SARS) in Guangdong province.

The virus was confirmed as a member of the Betacoronavirus subgroup and was named SARS-CoV[16]. On the thirteenth June, 2012, the first reported case of Middle East respiratory syndrome coronavirus (MERS-CoV) occurred in Jeddah, Saudi Arabia and caused an endemic in Middle Eastern countries. At the end of 2019, a novel coronavirus wasdiscovered at Wuhan in China [17, 18]. This virus was reported to be a member of the group 2b of coronaviruses[19] .

The ICTV named the virus as SARS-CoV-2 due to it'sgenetic similarity to SARS and the disease was namedCovid-19 because of the year of the outbreak [20]. In total nine HCoV strains are now identified: 229E, OC43, B814, OC16, OC37 and OC48, SARS-CoV, MERS and SARS-CoV-2 [21]. HCoV-229E was isolated in 1966 from human embryonic kidney cells and has been adapted to several types of cells, including MRC5, cells widely used in virology laboratories. HCoV-OC43 was isolated in 1967 on culture of trachea after passages on mice brains to the line HRT18 (human rectal carcinoma). HCoV-NL63 (strain Amsterdam 1) was isolated in 2004 from the LLC-MK2 line and SARS-CoV on Vero E6 cells [22]. Only HCoV-HKU1 to date has never been isolated in cell culture but it has been characterized by molecular biology. It is important to note that apart from the prototype strains, the coronavirus remain very difficult to cultivate and there are few isolates [23]. Finally, it is important to remember that these viruses are class 2 agents except the three SARS-CoV, which requirea level 3 containment laboratory for their handling. This literature review frommainpublications presents the genetics, the virulence factors, the etiology, epidemiology and pathophysiology of coronavirus diseases.

Genome similarity and conserved regions

The figure 2, 3, 4 and 5 represent the genome of *Coronaviridae*, the phylogenetic tree of *coronaviridae,* and *the* Human coronaviruses. The analysis of 33 full length publication papers and data GenBank analysis of all *coronaviridae* genome sequences and records howthat coronaviruses' genome is a linear, non-segmented single stranded, positive-sense RNA, directly infectious RNA molecule. The main characteristic of this virus is the size of its genome, which is the largest known viral RNA (27000 to 30 000 nucleotides). The genomic organization is conserved among all coronavirus species and approximately 20 000 nucleotides (nt) consist of two open reading frames ORF1a and ORF1b overlapping and encoding two protein precursors which are cleaved into 15 to 16 fragments and form the replication complex (Figure 2).

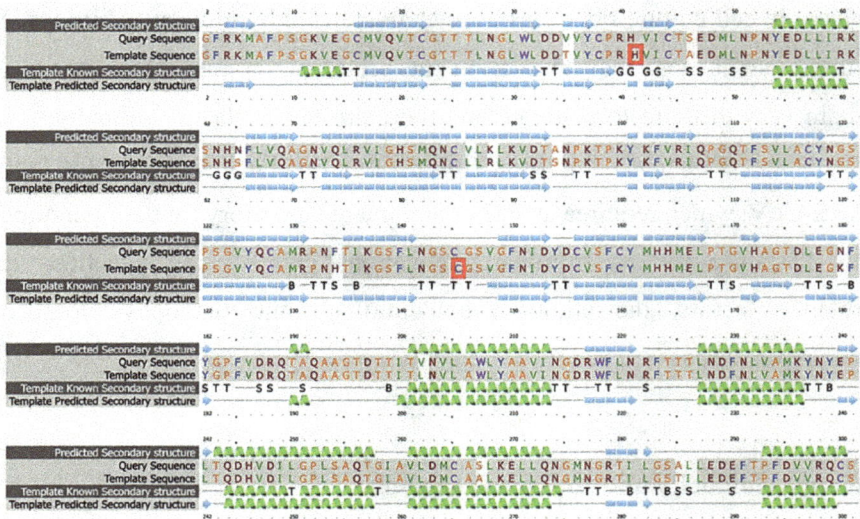

Figure 2: structure of coronaviridae genome (SARS-CoV 2) (Innophore technology).

The other conserved regions consist of four to five genes (HE-S-E-M-N) in a precise and conserved order and which encode the structural proteins. The figure 3 shows the phylogenic repartition among the human coronaviruses (HCoV) and show that the genome of the SARS-CoV-2 is mostly alike the previous human coronavirus (SARS-like bat CoV). Coronaviruses belong to *Coronaviridae* familly and fall into four distinct genera such us *alphacoronavirus* (1a, 1b) (blue), *betacoronavirus* (2a, 2b, 2c, 2d) (pink), *deltacoronavirus* (light green) and *gamma coronavirus* (deep green)[24, 25]. This tree is adapted from the published trees of Coronavirinae[26] wich was reconstructed with sequences of the complete RNA- dependent RNA polymerase-coding region of the representative novel coronaviruses (maximum likelihood method using MEGA 7.2 software). *Severe Acute respiratory syndrome coronavirus* (SARS-CoV) ; SARS- related coronavirus

(SARSr- CoV) ; the *Middle east respiratory syndrome coronavirus* (MERS-CoV) ; *Porcine entericdiarrhea virus* (PEDV) ; *Wuhan seafood market pneumonia* (Wuhan-Hu-1). Bat CoV RaTG13 Showed high sequence identity to SARS-CoV-2 [27].

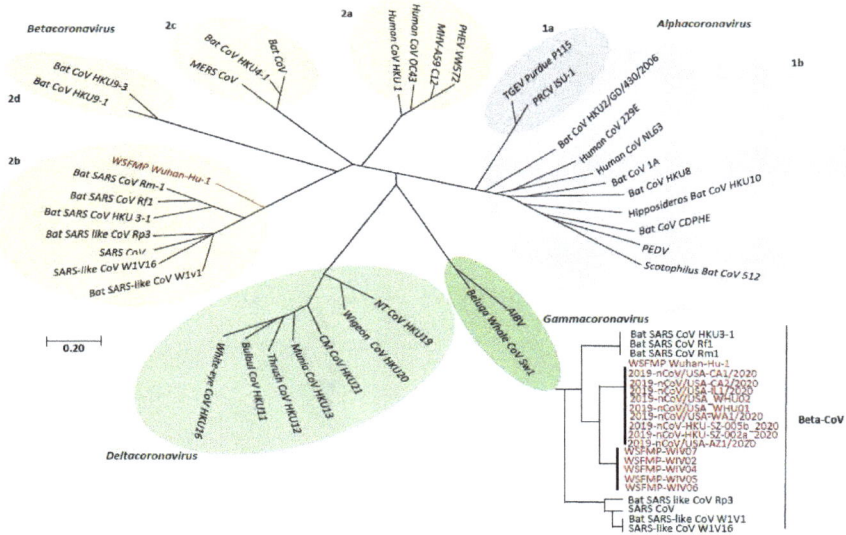

Figure 3: Evolutionary repartition of Coronaviridae (Adapted from [114]).

Figure 4 shows the evolutionary relation among the human coronaviruses (HCoV). The novel acute respiratory syndrome coronavirus 2 (SARS-CoV-2) is a new coronavirus that emergedthroughrecombination of bat SARS-relatedcoronaviruses (SARSr-CoVs) with infected civets and humans and adapted to these hosts and became pandemic[8].Middle eastrespiratory syndrome coronavirus (MERS-CoV) likelyspilled over from bats to dromedary. Figure 3: Evolutionary repartition of Coronaviridae (Adapted from [114]).

immunocompetent humans[13]. HKU1 and HCoV-OC43 are

alsomostlyharmless in humans[28].The coronaviruses infecting humans
(HCoVs) belong to alpha and beta coronaviruses genera. The alpha
coronaviruses infecting humans are HCoV-229E and HCoV NL63, and the
beta coronaviruses infecting humans are HCoV-HKU1, HCoV-OC43 (Figure
4). The Middle eastrespiratory syndrome coronavirus (MERS-CoV), SARS-
CoV and SARS-CoV-2 are betacoronaviruses[29] .

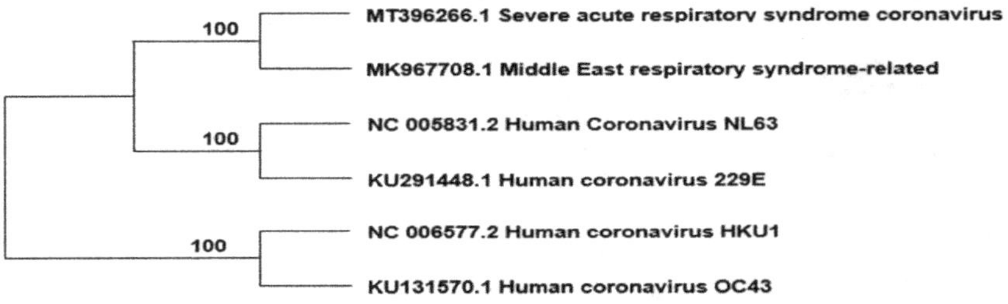

Figure 4: Evolutionary relationships of taxa of Human coronaviruses[103]

Coronavirus virulence factors

Figures 5 and 6 represent respectively the coronavirus structures, the host spectrum, the virulence factors similarity among HCoV and host factors. 6A show the similarity of Protein E, while 6B, 6C and 6D relate accordingly the similarity of Protein M, Protein S, and Protein N. Coronaviruses are enveloped pleomorphic viruses of 60 to 200 nm in diameter. The appearance in a crown visible by electron microscopy is due to the presence on the viral envelope of spicules in the shape of a club 20 nm high and made up of the surface protein S. The other envelope glycoproteins are the protein M, protein E and for group 2 coronavirus, hemagglutinin esterase (HE). The viral capsid is helical symmetry; it consists of the protein N, which is closely linked to genomic RNA. Protein S is a type I membrane glycoprotein, and plays a key role in the first stages of the viral cycle. It is responsible for the attachment of the virus to the target cell by its S1 subunit and largely determines the tissue tropism of the virus and its host spectrum. It is also responsible for the membrane fusion by its S2 subunit. In addition, it is the main target of the cellular and humoral immune response and induces the formation of neutralizing antibodies[29-34] .

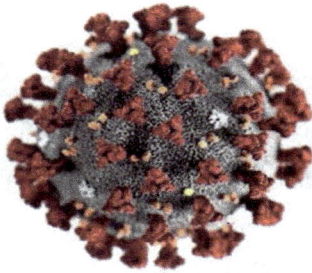
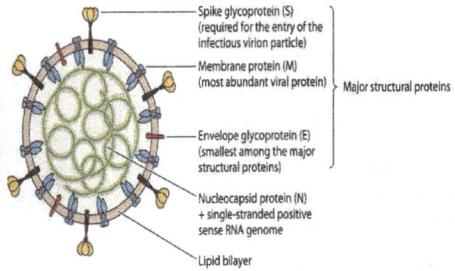

A   B

Figure 5: Structure of Coronaviridae (National Institute of Allergy and Infectious Diseases (NIAID), 2020. A : coronaviruses view in electronic microscope ; B : structure of coronaviruses.

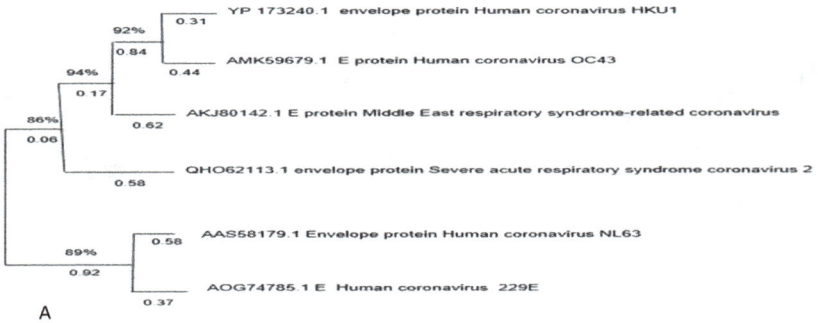

A

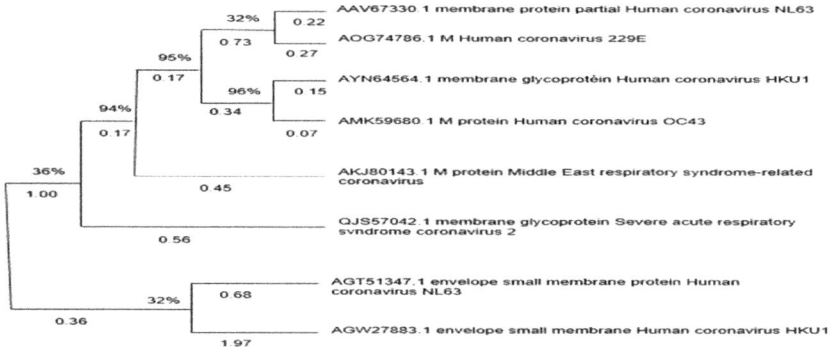

32% 0.22 AAV67330.1 membrane protein partial Human coronavirus NL63

0.73 AOG74786.1 M Human coronavirus 229E

95% 0.27

0.17 AYN64564.1 membrane glycoprotéin Human coronavirus HKU1

94% 96% 0.15

0.17 0.34 AMK59680.1 M protein Human coronavirus OC43

0.07

36% AKJ80143.1 M protein Middle East respiratory syndrome-related coronavirus

1.00 0.45

QJS57042.1 membrane glycoprotein Severe acute respiratory syndrome coronavirus 2

0.56

AGT51347.1 envelope small membrane protein Human coronavirus NL63

32% 0.68

0.36 AGW27883.1 envelope small membrane Human coronavirus HKU1

1.97

B

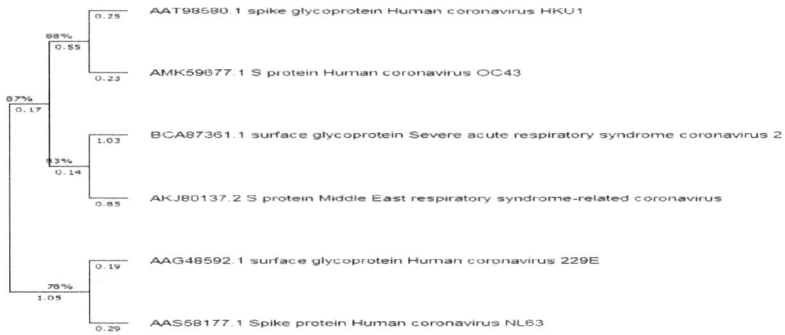

0.25 AAT98580.1 spike glycoprotein Human coronavirus HKU1

88%
0.55

0.23 AMK59877.1 S protein Human coronavirus OC43

87%
0.17

1.03 BCA87361.1 surface glycoprotein Severe acute respiratory syndrome coronavirus 2

83%
0.14

0.85 AKJ80137.2 S protein Middle East respiratory syndrome-related coronavirus

0.19 AAG48592.1 surface glycoprotein Human coronavirus 229E

78%
1.05

0.29 AAS58177.1 Spike protein Human coronavirus NL63

C

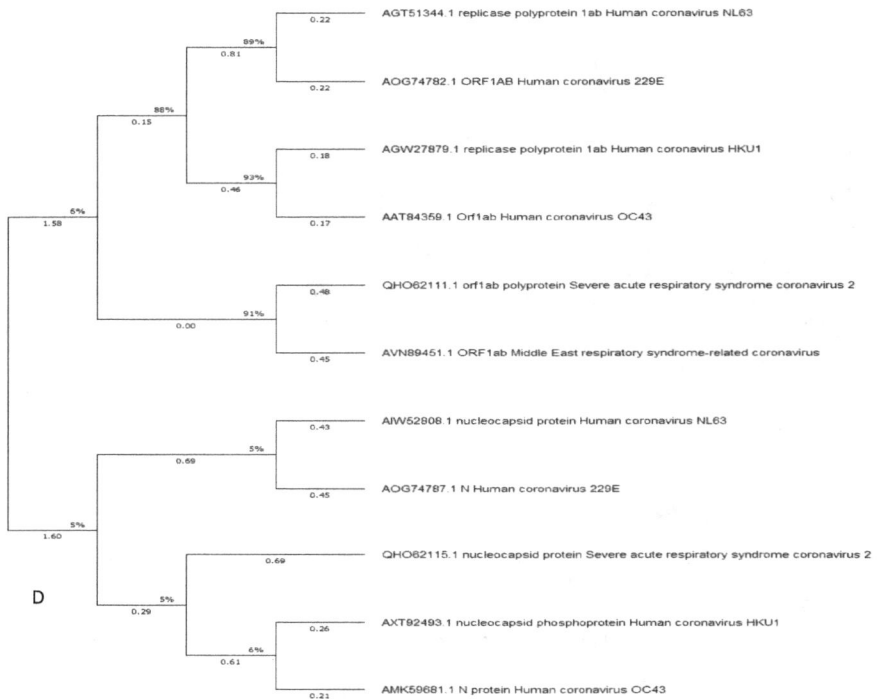

```
                                            ┌─ 0.22    AGT51344.1 replicase polyprotein 1ab Human coronavirus NL63
                                99%
                                0.81
                                            └─ 0.22    AOG74782.1 ORF1AB Human coronavirus 229E
                    86%
                    0.15
                                            ┌─ 0.18    AGW27879.1 replicase polyprotein 1ab Human coronavirus HKU1
                                93%
                                0.46
         6%                                 └─ 0.17    AAT84359.1 Orf1ab Human coronavirus OC43
         1.58
                                            ┌─ 0.48    QHO62111.1 orf1ab polyprotein Severe acute respiratory syndrome coronavirus 2
                                91%
                                0.00
                                            └─ 0.45    AVN89451.1 ORF1ab Middle East respiratory syndrome-related coronavirus

                                            ┌─ 0.43    AIW52808.1 nucleocapsid protein Human coronavirus NL63
                                5%
                                0.69
                                            └─ 0.45    AOG74787.1 N Human coronavirus 229E

         5%                                 ┌─ 0.69    QHO62115.1 nucleocapsid protein Severe acute respiratory syndrome coronavirus 2
         1.60
D                           5%
                            0.29            ┌─ 0.26    AXT92493.1 nucleocapsid phosphoprotein Human coronavirus HKU1
                                6%
                                0.61
                                            └─ 0.21    AMK59681.1 N protein Human coronavirus OC43
```

Figure 6: phylogenetical Analysis of HCoV Envelope (E), Spike (S), Membrane (M) and Nucleocapsid (N) protein. A : Similarity of Protein E, B: Similarity of Protein M, C : Similarity of Protein S, D : Similarity of Protein N.

Host factors

Figure 7 shows the host spectrum of the different coronavirus species. The species represented in blue are group 1 coronaviruses, those in red are group 2 coronaviruses and group 3 coronaviruses in black (aviancoronavirus). The arrows indicate the hypothetical crossing of monetary barriers with emerging success. Although human viruses, HCoVs have at some point emerged from an animal reservoir, with the original viruses being chiropterans (HCoV-229E, HCoV-NL63) or rodents (HCoV-OC43, HCoV-HKUl), with the putative intermediate hosts being cattle for HCoV-OC43 and camelids for HCoV-22928[28]. In addition Malnutrition has been reported as a virulence factor for the SARS-CoV-2 infection. The malnutrition (hyponutrition and hypernutrition) is associated with immune dysfunction. The hyponutrition which is mainlyproteindeficiency is associated with lowimmunoreactivitythat lead to T cellfunctionreduction, induction of IL4 and IL10 production, vitamins (A, B, D and E) deficiencies, hence the anaemia and micronutriment deficiencies. These conditions are surelyassocieted with increased SARS-CoV-2 virulence.

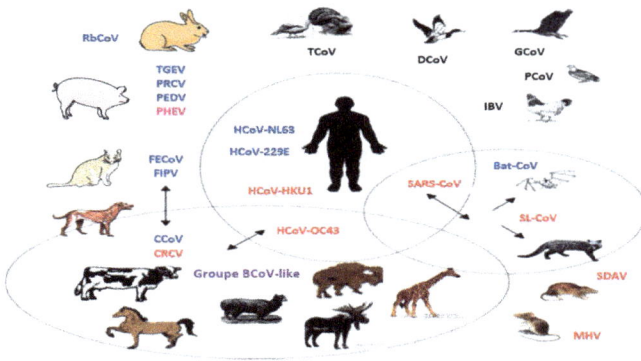

Figure 7: Host spectrum of different coronavirus species. Group 1 coronaviruses are written in blue, group 2 coronavruses in red, and group 3 coronaviruses (aviancoronaviruses) in black. The arrows indicate the hypothetical crossing of cash barriers with emergent success.

The hypernutrition which is essentialy do to sedentarism has the reverse effect. The immune dysregulation that exists in malnutrition and obesity can ahance the susceptibility to SARS-CoV-2 infection (figure 8)[35-37]. Malnourished people may have an immune deficiency to adequatelyfightagainst the virus. Malnourishedindividualsmaybe more susceptible to SARS-CoV-2 infection. Nutritional support is there for vital in severe Covid-19 patients[36]. The most relevant co-factor of SARS-CoV-2 is immune disfunction. Alsoolderage, comorbid conditions and polipharmacotherapy are the essential factors that increased the disease susceptibility.

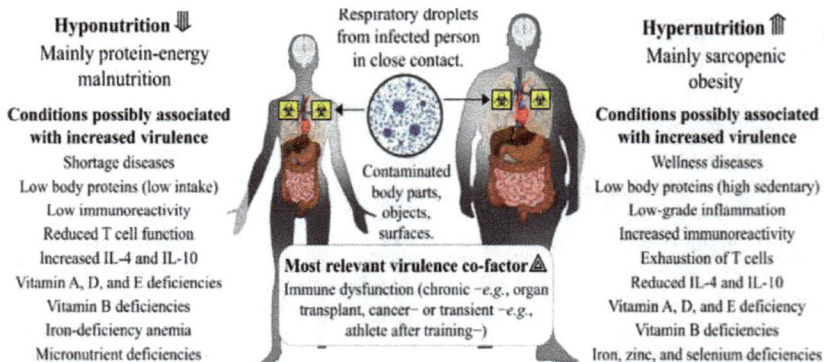

Hyponutrition ⇊
Mainly protein-energy malnutrition

Conditions possibly associated with increased virulence
Shortage diseases
Low body proteins (low intake)
Low immunoreactivity
Reduced T cell function
Increased IL-4 and IL-10
Vitamin A, D, and E deficiencies
Vitamin B deficiencies
Iron-deficiency anemia
Micronutrient deficiencies

Respiratory droplets from infected person in close contact.

Contaminated body parts, objects, surfaces.

Most relevant virulence co-factor ⚠
Immune dysfunction (chronic –e.g., organ transplant, cancer– or transient –e.g., athlete after training–)

Hypernutrition 🏛
Mainly sarcopenic obesity

Conditions possibly associated with increased virulence
Wellness diseases
Low body proteins (high sedentary)
Low-grade inflammation
Increased immunoreactivity
Exhaustion of T cells
Reduced IL-4 and IL-10
Vitamin A, D, and E deficiency
Vitamin B deficiencies
Iron, zinc, and selenium deficiencies

Figure 8: Malnutrition as virulence factor to coronavirus disease 2019 (Adapted from [115]).

Pathophysiology

The pathophysiology of HCoVis linked to the function of both the *nsp* and the structural proteins. Some studiesunderlined that *nsp*areable to block the host innate immune response [38]. Coronaviruses starting thesynthesis of polyprotein

1a/1ab (pp1a/pp1ab) in the host[16, 39] , of both pp1a and pp1ab polypeptides that are processed by virally encoded chymotrypsin-like protease (3CLpro) or main protease (*Mpro*), as well as one or two papain-like proteases for producing 16 non-structural proteins (*nsp*)[40] . In addition, other ORFs encode structural proteins, such as spike, membrane, envelope, nucleocapsid proteinsand accessory protein chains [41-43] .

Non structural protein 1 (Nsp1) fromsevere acute respiratory syndrome coronavirus suppresses host cell protein synthesis by binding to the 40S ribosomal subunit and endonucleolytically cleaving host mRNA[44]. This slows down translation in the infected cells and prevents, the proper expression of host factors that may be involved in the fight against the virus and its subsequent clearance by the innate immune. While Nsp1 prevents the expression of host proteins, viral protein synthesis continues unimpeded[45].

The function of nsp2 is not fullyunderstood. It is thought tobeassociate with the host endosome and host cellstability[46]. It is reported to be one of the conservedproteins of coronavirusesplaya key rolein viralreplication in culture. Nsp2 and nsp3 of SARS-CoV are detected not only as mature processedproteins but also as precursors of nsp1 and nsp3, which conferredthem a role as precursors in replication. Theseresultssuggest that nsp2 maybe involved in the regulation of nsp1 and nsp3 fonctions[47].

It has been reported that nsp3, nsp4, and nsp6 containtransmembranedomains and are likely to be involved in membrane anchoring of the replicationcomplex[48, 49].np3,alsoknown as papain-like protease (PLPro), is the largest non structural proteinencoded by the coronavirus (CoV) genome, with an averagemolecular mass of about 200 Kdand the second most promising vaccine candidate besides S protein[50]. It has differentdomainorganizationaccording to each*Coronavirus*genera.The nsp3 releases nsp1 and nsp2 frompolyproteins and interacts with not onlythe other viral nspsbut also RNA to form a replication/transcription complex. nsp3interacts with host protein translation to block host innateimmunity, promote cytokine expression and is alsoresponsible for the survival of the virus within the host by interfering with host proteins[51].nsp3 interact with nsp4 to playa key role in the replication of SARS-CoVinside the infected cells[52].Nsp6 alone has membrane proliferationproperties. As for Nsp5, it is a cysteineproteasewich is alsocalled, the main protease (Mpro). Nsp5 plays a major role in the virus replicationmakingMPro a potential and safetarget for anti-CoVdrug design. Nsp7 and nsp8 form an exadecamericcomplex. The bothact as RNA polymeraseprimase and forms a replicasecomplex for replication and transcription of the viral RNA genome[53]. It wasfound that there is an interconnection between the major nsp of SARS-CoV.Thus,nsp12 bound to nsp7/nsp8complex and play a central role in the viral replication[54]. It is the most conservedprotein in coronaviruses and an RNA-dependent RNA polymerase (RdRp)wich is the key enzyme in the viral replication/transcription complex. The nsp7/nsp8 complexincreases binding of nsp12 to RNA[55]. Nsp9 is a single-stranded RNA-binding proteinwich is alsoimplicated in the virus virulence. It ha been reported that nsp9 alsointeract with Nsp7/Nsp8 complex and is essential for the viral replication and potencialtarget of drugdevellopmentagainst the SARS-CoV-2[47]. Nsp10 is a small, single-domainproteinhaving 99% sequenceidentity with SARS-CoV Nsp10. Nsp10 acts as a scaffoldprotein to form the mRNA cap methylationcomplex with Nsp14 (exonuclease and N7-methyltransferase) and Nsp16 (2'-O-methyltransferase). It'sthere for a cofactor of nsp14 and nsp16 which enhancetheir activities[56].Nsp 13 is the 1 helicasesuperfamily withplays an essential role in viral replication and conservation across all CoV species[57].Nsp15 is a nidoviral RNA uridylate-specificendoribonuclease

(NendoU) belonging to EndoUenzymes family.firstly, nsp15 wasthought to be able to bind RNA and involved in viral replication, thenitwasshown that it'sratherresponsible for the proteininterference with the innate immune response.Otherstudies suggested that Nsp15 mediate the virus evasionof the host immune system.Recent data proved that this mechanism is not regulated by NendoUactivity[58, 59]. The Non-Structural Proteins (*nsp*) of *Coronavirus* and their biological functions are resumed in table 1.

Table 1 : Coronavirus non-structured proteins and their biological functions.

NAB nucleic acid binding, PL Pro papain-like protease, SUD SARS-unique domain, DMVs double-membrane vesicles, Mpro main protease, RdRp RNA-dependent RNA polymerase, MTasemethyltransferase, Exo N viral exoribonuclease, Nendo U viral endoribonuclease, , MDA5melanomadifferentiation associated protein 5, Ublubiquitin-like, Acacidic, 2'-O-MT 2'-O-methyltransferase, ADRP ADP-ribose-1'-phosphatase.

Protein	Functions
nsp1	Promotes cellular mRNA degradation and blocks host cell translation, results in blocking innate immune response
nsp2	No known function, binds to prohibiting proteins
nsp3	Large, multi-domain transmembrane protein, activities include
	• Ubl1 and Ac domains, interact with N protein
	ADRP activity, promotes cytokine expression
	PLPro/Deubiquitinase domain, cleaves viral polyprotein and blocks host innate immune response
	Ubl2, NAB, G2M, SUD, Y domains, unknown functions

Protein	Functions
nsp4	Potential transmembrane scaffold protein, important for proper structure of DMVs
nsp5	Mpro, cleaves viral polyprotein
nsp6	Potential transmembrane scaffold protein
nsp7	Forms hexadecameric complex with nsp8, may act as processivity clamp for RNA polymerase
nsp8	Forms hexadecameric complex with nsp7, may act as processivity clamp for RNA polymerase; may act as primase
nsp9	RNA binding protein
nsp10	Cofactor for nsp16 and nsp14, forms heterodimer with both and stimulates ExoN and 2-O-MT activity
nsp12	RdRp
nsp13	RNA helicase, 5′ triphosphatase
nsp14	N7 MTase and 3′-5′ exoribonuclease, ExoN; N7 MTase adds 5′ cap to viral RNAs, ExoN activity is important for proofreading of viral genome
nsp15	Viral endoribonuclease, NendoU
nsp16	2′-O-MT; shields viral RNA from MDA5 recognition

Epidemiology of coronavirus disease

In 2003, an epidemic of severe respiratory disease, severe acute respiratory syndrome (SARS), occurred in Guandong Province, China which quickly spread to other provinces in China. Intensive international research identified the new virus and see that it has the same morphological characteristics as and genetic characteristics of coronaviruses[60] and wascalled SARS-CoV. Recommendations for travel and measures to control the spread of the epidemic (rapid detection of cases, isolation, wearing of masks, etc.) were quickly issued by the WHO and quickly stopped the transmission of the virus [61, 62]. At the beginning of July 2003, no further transmission of the virus was observed and transmission was no longer observed and the WHO considered that the epidemia was contained. Some isolated cases, were identified between September 2003 and January 2004, with no other transmissions. It was then established that the natural host of the virus that causes SARS-CoV was a bat [63]. In 2012, Middle East Respiratory Syndrome Coronavirus (MERS-CoV) was identified in a patient with died of pneumonia in Saudi Arabia and a wave of severe pneumonia had occurred like previously in Jordan due to the same MERS-CoV[64]. Coronaviruses genetically very similar to MERS-CoV have been identified in bats that represent the virus reservoir. Humans become infected through contact with dromedaries, which are intermediate hosts.human-to-human transmission was not really established, the few cases observed were nosocomial infections[65].

The occurrence of severe pneumonia has been observed in December 2019 in the city of Wuhan, China. A new coronavirus associated with this outbreak was identified in early January 2020[66] and the disease, which emerged in 2019, was named Covid (**Corona**vi**r**us **d**isease)-19. The epidemic has spread rapidly outside China and all over the world. It is reported that the rapid emergence of SARS-CoV-2 and its pandemic spread are a proof that this virus is far more contagious than SARS-CoV-1 and MERS-CoV[26].

From MERS-CoV to SARS-CoV-2, the transmission has been identified as airborne droplet transmission[67].The human coronavirus infection's incubation periods are short. It is around three days for conventional CoV (HCoV-229E and HCoV-OC43), two to ten days for SARS-CoV (SARS-CoV and MERS – CoV) and two to fourteenth days for SARS-CoV-2[68] (Table 2).

The duration of the viral excretion in the respiratory tract is less well known, the RNA of conventional HCoV is detectable for about 14 days in the respiratory tract [69, 70]. SARS-CoV RNA can be detected by reverse transcriptase – polymerase chain reaction (RT-PCR) in the patient's respiratory secretions, stool, and urine up to approximately 30 days after the onset of the clinical signs [71].

Table 2: Epidemiology of Human coronaviruses. ARE: acute respiratory illness, CoV: coronavirus, ILI "influenza-like illness", MERS "Middle East respiratory syndrome", SARS "severe acute respiratory syndrome.

Table 2: Epidemiology of Human coronaviruses. ARE: acute respiratory illness, CoV: coronavirus, ILI "influenza-like illness", MERS "Middle East respiratory syndrome", SARS "severe acute respiratory syndrome."

	SARS-CoV 2	MERS-CoV	SRAS-Cov1	HCoV-HKU1	HCoV-NL63	HCoV-229E	HCoV-OC43
Discovery	2019	2012	2004	2004	2003	1960	1960
Source of infection for humans	-	Dromedaries, human	leather mouse, crawling cats, human	human	human	human	human
Transmission	Airborne droplet	Airborne droplet	Airborne droplet	Airborne droplet	Airborne droplet	Airborne droplet	Airborne droplet
Infection period	-	Spring	Spring	Winter - Spring	Winter - Spring	Winter Spring	Winter - Spring
Focus of geographic distribution	Worldwide	Arabian Peninsula	No more human cases since 2004 (previously East Asia)	Worldwide	Worldwide	Worldwide	Worldwide
Typical clinic	Viral pneumonia	Viral pneumonia	Viral pneumonia	ARE, ILI	ARE, ILI	ARE, ILI	ARE, ILI
Case fatality rate (CFR)	~ 7.1%[a]	-	9.6–11%	-	-	-	-
Incubation time	2–14 days	2–7 days	2–7 days	2-3 days	2-3 days	2-3 days	2-3 days

Genome similarity and conserved regions

The size of the genome and the complexity of the replication mode of coronaviruses granted them a high evolutionary potential.

The two major modes of evolution of coronaviruses are mutations and recombination [37, 72]. The mutation is due to an RNA dependent RNA-polymerase (RdRp), devoid of error correction system and generating many mutants replicates of RNA genomic. As with all RNA viruses, the viral population is heterogeneous and has a distribution in quasi-species. This distribution can be seen as an optimization strategy, being a structure allowing having a reservoir of variants with the capacities to cope with environmental changes.

It has been described for several coronaviruses not only in the context of persistent infections, but also in acute infections [73-76]. The best-known example is the emergence of respiratory porcine coronavirus (PRCV) in the 1980s, which is a spontaneous variant (deletion of 672 nucleotides (224 amino acids) in the gene encoding the protein S1) of enteric porcine coronavirus (TGEV). One of the biological consequences of this great deletion is the change in the tropism of the virus, from the TGEV to respiratory for PRCV[77].

The other evolutionary mode of coronaviruses is genetic recombination. This phenomenon is frequent in positive RNA viruses and seems to be favored in coronaviruses by the discontinuous mode of transcription. Recombination is the exchange of genetic material, which can be homologous if it takes place between two coronaviruses genomes, or heterologous if it involves other viral or cellular genes. Many recombinant forms have been described *in vitro* and *in vivo* in coronaviruses.

For example, feline coronavirus type II is the result of a double recombination between feline coronavirus type I and canine coronavirus, following a crossing of a species barrier in the dog-cat direction [78]. The important evolutionary capacity of coronaviruses was highlighted by the emergence of SARS-CoV[79]. The complete sequencing of HCoV-OC43 genome in 2005 by Vijgen*et al.* has further shown that this coronavirus is very close to bovine coronavirus, with more than 90% of nucleotide identity and on the other hand the E gene would have been acquired following a recombination with the porcine coronavirus of group 2 and hemagglutination encephalitis virus (HEV)[12, 80]. These data strongly suggest an emergence of HCoV-OC43 in the human population, secondary to an interspecies transmission in the bovine - human sense, which would have occurred at the end of the XIXth century[81, 82].

Several coronaviruses belonging to group 2a and with the same molecular lineage as HCoV-OC43 and BCoV have been recently described in elk, buffalo, giraffe, horse, and dog [83, 84]. It therefore seems that this group 2a "BCoV-like" coronavirus has a very broad host spectrum in wild and farmed mammals and has a high potential for interspecific passage [85]. Otherwise, the comparison of SL-CoV genomes from civets with the human SARS-CoV sequences shows approximately 30 000 nucleotides (a total of 212 positions of variation) of which 209 in a protein coding region (73 of these 209 are silent) [85, 86].

The SARS-CoV sequences of the early period (November 2002 to January 2003) are close to the SL-CoV sequences of civets, in particular the existence of a sequence of 29 nucleotides located at the level of ORF8, which has then disappeared when the virus adapted to humans (deletion of 29 nucleotides) [65, 87]. During the evolution of SARS-CoV, the mutation of amino acid residue 487 (from serine in civets to threonine in humans) of protein S seems to have contributed significantly to the adaptation of SARS-CoV to the human receptor angiotensin-converting enzyme 2 (ACE2) [88-90]. The percentage of similarity of sequences in six bat SL-CoV genomes has shown 89 to 90%, and around 87 to 92% with the civet sequences SL-CoV and SARS-CoV. The most variable regions are the S gene (76 –78% similarity) and ORF8.

The 29 nt region found in SL-CoV civets and early stage human strains is also found in SL-CoV bat [91]. Sequence analysis of SARS-CoV-2 has shown a typical structure to other coronavirus and its genome has been linkedto a previously identified coronavirus strain, SARS-CoV that caused the SARS outbreak in 2003 [92]. Structurally, the SARS coronavirus (SARS-CoV) has a well-defined composition comprising 14 binding residues that directly interact with human ACE2. Of these amino acids, eight have been conserved in SARS-CoV-2 [93].

Although the exact pathophysiological mechanisms underlying the emergence of SARS-CoV-2 are unknown, genomic similarities to SARS-CoV could help to explain the resulting inflammatory response that may lead to the onset of severe pneumonia [94].

The HCoV structure has shown that thereare most surface proteins, which havehypervariable regions, allowing it to escape immune pressure and, if necessary, to be able to enlarge its cellular tropism. Protein S of coronaviruses has a weak hemagglutination activity and binds to sialic acids. However, entry into target cells appears to require interaction with a specific protein receptor. Thus, cellular receptors are identified for somecoronaviruses: CEACAM1 molecule for the MHV, aminopeptidase N (APN) or CD13 for several group 1 coronaviruses (HCoV-229E, TGEV and PRCV, canine coronavirus and felines), the ACE2 molecule for HCoV-NL63 and SARS-CoV[63, 95] . The interactions between the protein S and its receptor seems complex and a large amount of data remains misunderstood.

The site of binding of the protein S to its receptor (receptor binding domain [RBD]) is located in different regions of the protein depending on the species of coronavirus, and itscleavage intoits two subunits S1 and S2 is variable, depending on the coronavirus and the cell type[96] . Some experimental data are unexpected: despite the amino acid sequences conserved at the level of the S1 protein of HCoV-229E and HCoV-NL63, these two human coronaviruses use different receptors (APN and ACE2, respectively). Furthermore, SARS-CoV uses the same cellular receptor as HCoV-NL63 while the S1 sequences are far apart;however, the RBD of the two viruses seems to be close and absent in SL-CoV.

The hypothesis is posed of an acquisition of this domain by recombination between SARS-CoV and another coronavirus close to HCoV-NL63 during its evolution in humans [97, 98]. The apparent plasticity of protein S and RBD would allow coronaviruses to adapt to different protein receptors or to heterologous receptors in different species and would be an advantage in emerging in new hosts. Group 2a coronaviruses are characterized by the existence of an HE protein, which forms a double row of small spicules of five nm high on the surface of the virus. It is a dimeric protein with hemagglutination activity and acetyl esterase. The gene encoding this protein is characteristic of group 2a CoVs. However, its expression is very variable.

Thus, in most MHV isolates, mutations, deletions or insertions have led to the loss of the open reading frameof this gene. Among the human coronaviruses, only the HCoV-OC43 and HCoV-HKU1 strains have the gene encoding HE[99, 100]. There is approximately 28% homology between the HEF surface protein of influenza C virus and the HE protein of HCoV-OC43 and bovine coronaviruses (BCoV).

Since the influenza C and HCoV-OC43 viruses infect the same tissues in humans, this homology suggests the acquisition of this gene by recombination. It should be noted that the HEF protein of the Influenza C virus has a membrane fusion activity, which is absent in the HE protein of CoV[101, 102]. This protein recognizes cell receptors containing acetylated 9-O sialic acids and induces the formation of neutralizing antibodies. Thus, it would have a function of attachment protein and of initiation of the infection, additive to that of protein S. However, its main function would be the acetyl-esterase activity. Many questions exist about the *in vivo* course of the first stages of the replication cycle for Group 2a CoVs. The HE protein required little attention, probably because it would not be present in the CoVs most studied so far (IBV, MHV, TGEV, SARS- CoV, HCoV-229E and HCoV-NL63) [103, 104]. For all Group 2a CoVs studied so far, the binding of protein S to a sialic acid corresponds with the preferential substrate of HE. The HE protein would therefore allow optimal use of sialic acids as attachment factors.

The mode of entry of CoV expressing the HE protein would then be close to that adopted by the influenza A and B viruses, and the functional balance described between hemagglutinin and neuraminidase HA/NA could also exist between S and HE [85]. Protein S is the factor that determines the host spectrum and tissue tropism of coronavirus strains and is the carrier where the differences between HCoV, BCoV and civet coronavirus are concentrated[82]. Cellular protein receptors, in addition to binding to sialic acids have been described for a number of coronaviruses. However, some coronavirus, such as BCoV and HCoV-OC43, use only a sialic acid as the same used by the influenza C virus.

Epidemiology transmission of HCoV occurs mainly directly through droplets of oropharyngeal secretions dispersed by the cough of an infected or symptomatic person. During SARS, MERS and Covid-19, those infected aremainly person who had close contact with a positive case. Airborne viral spread appears to be infrequent as well as indirect "hand-carried" transmission. However, these transmission routes must be taken into account for the control of epidemics, especially in healthcare settings.

Studies of "survival" or maintenance of pathogenicity in air is rare and difficult. The number of secondary cases from index case was only studied within the framework of SARS in 2003. This virus is moderately contagious, with an average number of secondary cases estimated at 2.2 to 3.6. However, super-propagation events with several dozen secondary cases have been described, and have played an important role in the spread of the disease[105].

Concerning old outbreak of the human coronaviruses, among the classic coronavirus strains isolated in the 1960s, only HCoV-229E and HCoV-OC43 were studied and maintained in culture [106]. These studies have shown that HCoV represents a group of respiratory pathogens that infectsall age groups and involvesin lower respiratory infections (bronchitis, bronchiolitis, pneumonitis, exacerbations of asthma)[107]. The primary infections occur in the early years and re-infections are common throughout life. These reinfections are symptomatic in approximately 45% of cases. The infection rate is relatively uniform across all age groups.

This situation differs from other observed for respiratory viruses such as respiratory syncytial virus (RSV), for which infection rates decrease with age. The classic coronaviruses circulate in an epidemic mode, most often between January and May in areas with a temperate climate. The cyclical and alternative nature of HCoV-229E and HCoV-OC43 strains had been stressed as well as the probable existence of other serotypes. That suggested the combined use of several serological techniques such as complement fixation, inhibition of hemagglutination and sero-neutralization[80].

Regarding HCoV-NL63 and HCoV-HKU1, their recent identification reflects a reduced number of epidemiological data. HCoV-NL63 is a group 1 coronavirus that was discovered and identified by molecular techniques from a respiratory sample of a seven-month-old infant hospitalized for bronchiolitis in January 2003 and the prototype strain was called Amsterdam 1[95]. The retrospective studies have shown that HCoV-NL63 is not an emerging virus but a virus already circulating in the human population and newly identified[108].

HCoV-HKU1 is a group 2a coronavirus, discovered in Hong Kong in 2005, in a 71-year-old patient hospitalized for pneumonia. This virus has been characterized on a molecular level and determined three different genotypes; A, B, and C of HCoV-HKU1, genotype C being a recombinant of genotypes A and B. In addition, this virus is not responsible for a new disease, only its knowledge is emerging [109]. HCoV-HKU1 has not been adapted to cell culture.

In 2006 and 2007, some studies were published on the circulation of the four HCoVs (HCoV-229E, HCoV-OC43, HCoV-NL63 and HCoV-HKU1). These studies have nonetheless confirmed the epidemic nature of human coronavirus infections, at the winter – spring junction (peak in February). The four HCoV co-circulate with variations in the distribution of different species according to geography and years[110]. SARS is a special story in coronavirus infections.

According to the WHO, on March 12th, 2003, SARS-CoV made about 8000 probable cases and 800 deaths were declared, the great majority in China. The estimated fatality rate is 0% for subjects under 35 years of age, 7% for subjects 35 to 65 years of age, and 47% for subjects over 65 years of age. WHO declared the end of human-to-human transmission in July 2003[8]. Since July 2003, several cases of laboratory contamination have been reported in Asia; finally, epidemiological reports from the Guangdong Center for Disease Control and Prevention have indicatedthat in January 2004, six months after the end of the epidemic, four patients were hospitalized for a mild SARS-CoV infection. The molecular study of these strains concluded that they derived from the same source as the epidemic strains from 2002 to 2003 [8, 95].

MERS-CoV triggered an occurrence of respiratory illness in the Middle East with secondary spread to Europe, Africa, Asia, and North America. The diseases occurred mainly in the Middle East states with highest cases of 88% followed by 11% in Asia, 0.8% in Europe, 0.1% in Africa and 0.1% in USA. The age group with highest risk for acquiring as primary cases of infections is 50-59 years and high risk for acquiring as secondary cases of infections is 30-39 years. The total number of associated fatality rate is 858 (34.40%) [111].

Recent coronavirus outbreak was due to a novel SARS-CoV-2 coronavirus. In December 2019, reports of pneumonia-like conditions came in Wuhan, China. The viral spillover is believed to happen in a seafood market in Wuhan, Hubei Province, China [112]. WHO declared Covid-19 to be a public health emergency of international concern (PHEIC) on 30th January 2020[113].

Contributors

Christèle T. Nguepou[1], Essoham Ataba[1], Banfitebiyi Gambogou[2], Manuel Ritter[3], Eya H. Kamassa[1], Fagdéba D. Bara[1], Simplice D. Karou[1]

[1]Advanced School of Biological and Food Techniques (ESTBA) / Laboratory of Microbiology and Food Quality Control / Research Unit in Immunology and Immunomodulation (UR2IM), University of Lomé, Togo.

[2]Togolese Institute for Agronomic Research (ITRA), Togo.

[3]Institute for Medical Microbiology, Immunology and Parasitology (IMMIP), University Hospital Bonn, Germany.

REFERENCES

1.   Katawa G, Layland LE, Debrah AY, et al. Hyperreactive onchocerciasis is characterized by a combination of Th17-Th2 immune responses and reduced regulatory T cells. *PLoS Negl Trop Dis*. Jan 2015;9(1):e3414. doi:10.1371/journal.pntd.0003414

2.   Katawa G, Kolou M, Nadjir LK, Ataba E, Bomboma G, Karou SD. CD4 T-Lymphocytes Count in HIV-Toxoplasma gondii Co-Infected Pregnant Women Undergoing a Prevention of Mother-to-Child Transmission Program. *Journal of Biosciences and Medicines*. 2018;6(04):76.doi: 10.4236/jbm.2018.64006

3.   Nadjir LK, Kolou M, Katawa G, et al. Seroprevalence of hepatitis B virus, hepatitis C virus, and human immunodeficiency virus among volunteer blood donors in the National Blood Transfusion Center of Lom. *Int J Blood Transfus Immunohematol*. 2017;7:41-45. doi:10.5348/ijbti-2017-33-OA-6

4.   Kolou M, Katawa G, Salou M, et al. High Prevalence of Hepatitis B Virus Infection in the Age Range of 20-39 Years Old Individuals in Lome. *Open Virol J*. 2017;11:1-7. doi:10.2174/1874357901710011001

5.   Tchopba CN, Ataba E, Katawa G, et al. COVID-19: epidemiology, pathogenesis and immununological basis. *Al-Nahrain Journal of Science*. 2020;(4):1-12. doi:10.22401/ANJS.00.4.01

6.   Chen Y, Liu Q, Guo D. Emerging coronaviruses: Genome structure, replication, and pathogenesis. *J Med Virol*. Oct 2020;92(10):2249. doi:10.1002/jmv.26234

7.   Kaushik S, Sharma Y, Kumar R, Yadav JP. The Indian perspective of COVID-19 outbreak. *Virusdisease*. May 2020:1-8. doi:10.1007/s13337-020-00587-x

8.   Adachi S, Koma T, Doi N, Nomaguchi M, Adachi A. Commentary: Origin and evolution of pathogenic coronaviruses. *Front Immunol*. 2020;11:811. doi:10.3389/fimmu.2020.00811

9.   Woo PC, Lau SK, Huang Y, Yuen KY. Coronavirus diversity, phylogeny and interspecies jumping. *Exp Biol Med (Maywood)*. Oct 2009;234(10):1117-27. doi:10.3181/0903-MR-94

10.   Belouzard S, Millet JK, Licitra BN, Whittaker GR. Mechanisms of coronavirus cell entry mediated by the viral spike protein. *Viruses*. 06 2012;4(6):1011-33. doi:10.3390/v4061011

11.   Niu J, Shen L, Huang B, et al. Non-invasive bioluminescence imaging of HCoV-OC43 infection and therapy in the central nervous system of live mice. *Antiviral Res*. 01 2020;173:104646. doi:10.1016/j.antiviral.2019.104646

12.   Lau SK, Lee P, Tsang AK, et al. Molecular epidemiology of human coronavirus OC43 reveals evolution of different genotypes over time and recent emergence of a novel genotype due to natural recombination. *J Virol*. Nov 2011;85(21):11325-37. doi:10.1128/JVI.05512-11

13.   Huynh J, Li S, Yount B, et al. Evidence supporting a zoonotic origin of human coronavirus strain NL63. *J Virol*. Dec 2012;86(23):12816-25. doi:10.1128/JVI.00906-12

14.   Oong XY, Ng KT, Takebe Y, et al. Identification and evolutionary dynamics of two novel human coronavirus OC43 genotypes associated with acute respiratory infections: phylogenetic, spatiotemporal and transmission network analyses. *Emerg Microbes Infect*. Jan 2017;6(1):e3. doi:10.1038/emi.2016.132

15.   Haake C, Cook S, Pusterla N, Murphy B. Coronavirus Infections in Companion Animals: Virology, Epidemiology, Clinical and Pathologic Features. *Viruses*. 09 2020;12(9).doi:10.3390/v12091023

16.   Vabret AD, J. Brison, E. Brouard, J. Freymuth, F. . Coronavirus humains (HCoV). *Pathologie Biologie*. 2009;(57):149–160. doi:10.1016/j.patbio.2008.02.018

17.   Jin Y, Song JR, Xie ZP, et al. Prevalence and clinical characteristics of human CoV-HKU1 in children with acute respiratory tract infections in China. *J Clin Virol*. Oct 2010;49(2):126-30. doi:10.1016/j.jcv.2010.07.002

18.   Mallah SI, Ghorab OK, Al-Salmi S, et al. COVID-19: breaking down a global health crisis. *Ann Clin Microbiol Antimicrob*. May 2021;20(1):35. doi:10.1186/s12941-021-00438-7

19.   Chu DKW, Pan Y, Cheng SMS, et al. Molecular Diagnosis of a Novel Coronavirus (2019-nCoV) Causing an Outbreak of Pneumonia. *Clin Chem.* 04 2020;66(4):549-555. doi:10.1093/clinchem/hvaa029

20.   Lu R, Zhao X, Li J, et al. Genomic characterisation and epidemiology of 2019 novel coronavirus: implications for virus origins and receptor binding. *Lancet.* 02 2020;395(10224):565-574. doi:10.1016/S0140-6736(20)30251-8

21.   Singh DD, Han I, Choi EH, Yadav DK. Recent Advances in Pathophysiology, Drug Development and Future Perspectives of SARS-CoV-2. *Front Cell Dev Biol.* 2020;8:580202. doi:10.3389/fcell.2020.580202

22.   Song X, Shi Y, Ding W, et al. Cryo-EM analysis of the HCoV-229E spike glycoprotein reveals dynamic prefusion conformational changes. *Nat Commun.* 01 2021;12(1):141. doi:10.1038/s41467-020-20401-y

23.   Nascimento Júnior JAC, Santos AM, Cavalcante RCM, et al. Mapping the technological landscape of SARS, MERS, and SARS-CoV-2 vaccines. *Drug Dev Ind Pharm.* Apr 2021;47(4):673-684. doi:10.1080/03639045.2021.1908343

24.   Graham RL, Donaldson EF, Baric RS. A decade after SARS: strategies for controlling emerging coronaviruses. *Nat Rev Microbiol.* Dec 2013;11(12):836-48. doi:10.1038/nrmicro3143

25.   Drexler JF, Corman VM, Drosten C. Ecology, evolution and classification of bat coronaviruses in the aftermath of SARS. *Antiviral Res.* Jan 2014;101:45-56. doi:10.1016/j.antiviral.2013.10.013

26.   Chung Y-S, Kim JM, Man Kim H, et al. Genetic Characterization of Middle East Respiratory Syndrome Coronavirus, South Korea, 2018. *Emerging infectious diseases.* 2019;25(5):958-962. doi:10.3201/eid2505.181534

27.   Zhou P, Yang X-L, Wang X-G, et al. Discovery of a novel coronavirus associated with the recent pneumonia outbreak in humans and its potential bat origin. *BioRxiv.* 2020.doi: 10.1038/s41586-020-2012-7

28. Corman VM, Muth D, Niemeyer D, Drosten C. Hosts and sources of endemic human coronaviruses. *Advances in virus research*. 2018;100:163-188.doi: 10.1016/bs.aivir.2018.01.001

29. Dai L, Gao GF. Viral targets for vaccines against COVID-19. *Nat Rev Immunol*. 02 2021;21(2):73-82. doi: 10.1038/s41577-020-00480-0.

30. Naydenova K, Muir KW, Wu LF, et al. Structure of the SARS-CoV-2 RNA-dependent RNA polymerase in the presence of favipiravir-RTP. *Proc Natl Acad Sci U S A*. 02 2021;118(7)doi:10.1073/pnas.2021946118. doi: 10.1073/pnas.2021946118

31. Oliveira SC, de Magalhães MTQ, Homan EJ. Immunoinformatic Analysis of SARS-CoV-2 Nucleocapsid Protein and Identification of COVID-19 Vaccine Targets. *Front Immunol*. 2020;11:587615. doi:10.3389/fimmu.2020.587615

32. Serrão VHB, Lee JE. FRETing over SARS-CoV-2: Conformational Dynamics of the Spike Glycoprotein. *Cell Host Microbe*. 12 2020;28(6):778-779. doi:10.1016/j.chom.2020.11.008

33. Srinivasan S, Cui H, Gao Z, et al. Structural Genomics of SARS-CoV-2 Indicates Evolutionary Conserved Functional Regions of Viral Proteins. *Viruses*. 03 2020;12(4). doi:10.3390/v12040360

34. Wrapp D, Wang N, Corbett KS, et al. Cryo-EM structure of the 2019-nCoV spike in the prefusion conformation. *Science*. 03 2020;367(6483):1260-1263. doi:10.1126/science.abb2507

35. Bhattacharya I, Ghayor C, Pérez Dominguez A, Weber FE. From Influenza Virus to Novel Corona Virus (SARS-CoV-2)-The Contribution of Obesity. *Front Endocrinol (Lausanne)*. 2020;11:556962. doi:10.3389/fendo.2020.556962

36. Almond MH, Edwards MR, Barclay WS, Johnston SL. Obesity and susceptibility to severe outcomes following respiratory viral infection. *Thorax*. Jul 2013;68(7):684-6. doi:10.1136/thoraxjnl-2012-203009

37.   Wang Y, Grunewald M, Perlman S. Coronaviruses: An Updated Overview of Their Replication and Pathogenesis. *Methods Mol Biol*. 2020;2203:1-29. doi:10.1007/978-1-0716-0900-2_1

38.   Fehr AR, Channappanavar R, Jankevicius G, et al. The Conserved Coronavirus Macrodomain Promotes Virulence and Suppresses the Innate Immune Response during Severe Acute Respiratory Syndrome Coronavirus Infection. *mBio*. 12 2016;7(6). doi:10.1128/mBio.01721-16

39.   Romano M, Ruggiero A, Squeglia F, Maga G, Berisio R. A Structural View of SARS-CoV-2 RNA Replication Machinery: RNA Synthesis, Proofreading and Final Capping. *Cells*. 05 2020;9(5). doi:10.3390/cells9051267

40.   Niemeyer D, Mösbauer K, Klein EM, et al. The papain-like protease determines a virulence trait that varies among members of the SARS-coronavirus species. *PLoS Pathog*. 09 2018;14(9):e1007296. doi:10.1371/journal.ppat.1007296

41.   Niu X, Kong F, Hou YJ, Wang Q. Crucial mutation in the exoribonuclease domain of nsp14 of PEDV leads to high genetic instability during viral replication. *Cell Biosci*. Jun 2021;11(1):106. doi:10.1186/s13578-021-00598-1

42.   Kindler E, Gil-Cruz C, Spanier J, et al. Early endonuclease-mediated evasion of RNA sensing ensures efficient coronavirus replication. *PLoS Pathog*. 02 2017;13(2):e1006195. doi:10.1371/journal.ppat.1006195

43.   Stodola JK, Dubois G, Le Coupanec A, Desforges M, Talbot PJ. The OC43 human coronavirus envelope protein is critical for infectious virus production and propagation in neuronal cells and is a determinant of neurovirulence and CNS pathology. *Virology*. 02 2018;515:134-149. doi:10.1016/j.virol.2017.12.023

44.   Nakagawa K, Makino S. Mechanisms of Coronavirus Nsp1-Mediated Control of Host and Viral Gene Expression. *Cells*. 02 2021;10(2). doi:10.3390/cells10020300

45.   Vann KR, Tencer AH, Kutateladze TG. Inhibition of translation and immune responses by the virulence factor Nsp1 of SARS-CoV-2. *Signal Transduct Target Ther.* 10 2020;5(1):234. doi:10.1038/s41392-020-00350-0

46.   Angeletti S, Benvenuto D, Bianchi M, Giovanetti M, Pascarella S, Ciccozzi M. COVID-2019: The role of the nsp2 and nsp3 in its pathogenesis. *J Med Virol.* 06 2020;92(6):584-588. doi:10.1002/jmv.25719

47.   Gorkhali R, Koirala P, Rijal S, Mainali A, Baral A, Bhattarai HK. Structure and Function of Major SARS-CoV-2 and SARS-CoV Proteins. *Bioinform Biol Insights.* 2021;15:11779322211025876. doi:10.1177/11779322211025876

48.   Oudshoorn D, Rijs K, Limpens RWAL, et al. Expression and Cleavage of Middle East Respiratory Syndrome Coronavirus nsp3-4 Polyprotein Induce the Formation of Double-Membrane Vesicles That Mimic Those Associated with Coronaviral RNA Replication. *mBio.* 11 2017;8(6). doi:10.1128/mBio.01658-17

49.   Angelini MM, Akhlaghpour M, Neuman BW, Buchmeier MJ. Severe acute respiratory syndrome coronavirus nonstructural proteins 3, 4, and 6 induce double-membrane vesicles. *mBio.* Aug 2013;4(4). doi:10.1128/mBio.00524-13

50.   Lei J, Kusov Y, Hilgenfeld R. Nsp3 of coronaviruses: Structures and functions of a large multi-domain protein. *Antiviral Res.* 01 2018;149:58-74. doi:10.1016/j.antiviral.2017.11.001

51.   Báez-Santos YM, St John SE, Mesecar AD. The SARS-coronavirus papain-like protease: structure, function and inhibition by designed antiviral compounds. *Antiviral Res.* Mar 2015;115:21-38. doi:10.1016/j.antiviral.2014.12.015

52.   Sakai Y, Kawachi K, Terada Y, Omori H, Matsuura Y, Kamitani W. Two-amino acids change in the nsp4 of SARS coronavirus abolishes viral replication. *Virology.* 10 2017;510:165-174. doi:10.1016/j.virol.2017.07.019

53.   Kirchdoerfer RN, Ward AB. Structure of the SARS-CoV nsp12 polymerase bound to nsp7 and nsp8 co-factors. *Nat Commun.* 05 2019;10(1):2342. doi:10.1038/s41467-019-10280-3

54.   te Velthuis AJ, Arnold JJ, Cameron CE, van den Worm SH, Snijder EJ. The RNA polymerase activity of SARS-coronavirus nsp12 is primer dependent. *Nucleic Acids Res.* Jan 2010;38(1):203-14. doi:10.1093/nar/gkp904

55.   Subissi L, Imbert I, Ferron F, et al. SARS-CoV ORF1b-encoded nonstructural proteins 12-16: replicative enzymes as antiviral targets. *Antiviral Res.* Jan 2014;101:122-30. doi:10.1016/j.antiviral.2013.11.006

56.   Mirza MU, Froeyen M. Structural elucidation of SARS-CoV-2 vital proteins: Computational methods reveal potential drug candidates against main protease, Nsp12 polymerase and Nsp13 helicase. *J Pharm Anal.* Aug 2020;10(4):320-328. doi:10.1016/j.jpha.2020.04.008

57.   Mickolajczyk KJ, Shelton PMM, Grasso M, et al. Force-dependent stimulation of RNA unwinding by SARS-CoV-2 nsp13 helicase. *Biophys J.* 03 2021;120(6):1020-1030. doi:10.1016/j.bpj.2020.11.2276

58.   Deng X, Hackbart M, Mettelman RC, et al. Coronavirus nonstructural protein 15 mediates evasion of dsRNA sensors and limits apoptosis in macrophages. *Proc Natl Acad Sci U S A.* 05 2017;114(21):E4251-E4260. doi:10.1073/pnas.1618310114

59.   Liu X, Fang P, Fang L, et al. Porcine deltacoronavirus nsp15 antagonizes interferon-β production independently of its endoribonuclease activity. *Mol Immunol.* 10 2019;114:100-107. doi:10.1016/j.molimm.2019.07.003

60.   Drosten C, Günther S, Preiser W, et al. Identification of a novel coronavirus in patients with severe acute respiratory syndrome. *N Engl J Med.* May 2003;348(20):1967-76. doi:10.1056/NEJMoa030747

61.   Seto WH, Tsang D, Yung RW, et al. Effectiveness of precautions against droplets and contact in prevention of nosocomial transmission of severe acute respiratory syndrome (SARS). *Lancet.* May 2003;361(9368):1519-20. doi:10.1016/s0140-6736(03)13168-6

62.   Zimmermann P, Curtis N. Coronavirus Infections in Children Including COVID-19: An Overview of the Epidemiology, Clinical Features, Diagnosis, Treatment and Prevention Options in Children. *Pediatr Infect Dis J*. 05 2020;39(5):355-368. doi:10.1097/INF.0000000000002660

63.   Yip CC, Lam CS, Luk HK, et al. A six-year descriptive epidemiological study of human coronavirus infections in hospitalized patients in Hong Kong. *Virol Sin*. Feb 2016;31(1):41-8. doi:10.1007/s12250-016-3714-8

64.   Zaki AM, van Boheemen S, Bestebroer TM, Osterhaus AD, Fouchier RA. Isolation of a novel coronavirus from a man with pneumonia in Saudi Arabia. *N Engl J Med*. Nov 2012;367(19):1814-20. doi:10.1056/NEJMoa1211721

65.   Jo WK, Drosten C, Drexler JF. The evolutionary dynamics of endemic human coronaviruses. *Virus Evol*. Jan 2021;7(1):veab020. doi:10.1093/ve/veab020

66.   Zhou P, Yang X-L, Wang X-G, et al. A pneumonia outbreak associated with a new coronavirus of probable bat origin. *nature*. 2020;579(7798):270-273. doi: 10.1038/s41586-020-2012-7.

67.   Shereen MA, Khan S, Kazmi A, Bashir N, Siddique R. COVID-19 infection: Origin, transmission, and characteristics of human coronaviruses. *J Adv Res*. Jul 2020;24:91-98. doi:10.1016/j.jare.2020.03.005

68.   Huang SH, Su MC, Tien N, et al. Epidemiology of human coronavirus NL63 infection among hospitalized patients with pneumonia in Taiwan. *J Microbiol Immunol Infect*. Dec 2017;50(6):763-770. doi:10.1016/j.jmii.2015.10.008

69.   Asghari A, Naseri M, Safari H, Saboory E, Parsamanesh N. The Novel Insight of SARS-CoV-2 Molecular Biology and Pathogenesis and Therapeutic Options. *DNA Cell Biol*. Oct 2020;39(10):1741-1753. doi:10.1089/dna.2020.5703

70.   Graepel KW, Lu X, Case JB, Sexton NR, Smith EC, Denison MR. Proofreading-Deficient Coronaviruses Adapt for Increased Fitness over Long-Term Passage without Reversion of Exoribonuclease-Inactivating Mutations. *mBio*. 11 2017;8(6). doi:10.1128/mBio.01503-17

71.   Beidas M, Chehadeh W. PCR array profiling of antiviral genes in human embryonic kidney cells expressing human coronavirus OC43 structural and accessory proteins. *Arch Virol.* Aug 2018;163(8):2065-2072. doi:10.1007/s00705-018-3832-8

72.   Viswanathan T, Arya S, Chan SH, et al. Structural Basis of RNA Cap Modification by SARS-CoV-2 Coronavirus. *bioRxiv.* Apr 2020. doi:10.1101/2020.04.26.061705

73.   Sola I, Mateos-Gomez PA, Almazan F, Zuñiga S, Enjuanes L. RNA-RNA and RNA-protein interactions in coronavirus replication and transcription. *RNA Biol.* 2011 Mar-Apr 2011;8(2):237-48. doi:10.4161/rna.8.2.14991

74.   Wu Z, Yang L, Ren X, et al. ORF8-Related Genetic Evidence for Chinese Horseshoe Bats as the Source of Human Severe Acute Respiratory Syndrome Coronavirus. *J Infect Dis.* Feb 2016;213(4):579-83. doi:10.1093/infdis/jiv476

75.   Uhler C, Shivashankar GV. Mechano-genomic regulation of coronaviruses and its interplay with ageing. *Nat Rev Mol Cell Biol.* 05 2020;21(5):247-248. doi:10.1038/s41580-020-0242-z

76.   Vishnubalaji R, Shaath H, Alajez NM. Protein Coding and Long Noncoding RNA (lncRNA) Transcriptional Landscape in SARS-CoV-2 Infected Bronchial Epithelial Cells Highlight a Role for Interferon and Inflammatory Response. *Genes (Basel).* 07 2020;11(7). doi:10.3390/genes11070760

77.   Cao Y, Li L, Feng Z, et al. Comparative genetic analysis of the novel coronavirus (2019-nCoV/SARS-CoV-2) receptor ACE2 in different populations. *Cell Discov.* 2020;6:11. doi:10.1038/s41421-020-0147-1

78.   Zella D, Giovanetti M, Cella E, et al. The importance of genomic analysis in cracking the coronavirus pandemic. *Expert Rev Mol Diagn.* Apr 2021:1-16. doi:10.1080/14737159.2021.1917998

79.   Sironi M, Hasnain SE, Rosenthal B, et al. SARS-CoV-2 and COVID-19: A genetic, epidemiological, and evolutionary perspective. *Infect Genet Evol.* Oct 2020;84:104384. doi:10.1016/j.meegid.2020.104384

80.   Kin N, Miszczak F, Diancourt L, et al. Comparative molecular epidemiology of two closely related coronaviruses, bovine coronavirus (BCoV) and human coronavirus OC43 (HCoV-OC43), reveals a different evolutionary pattern. *Infect Genet Evol*. 06 2016;40:186-191. doi:10.1016/j.meegid.2016.03.006

81.   Xiao J, Price J, Mina N. 1051: HUMAN CORONAVIRUS OC43-INDUCED ACUTE RESPIRATORY DISTRESS SYNDROME. *Critical Care Medicine*. 2018;46(1):509. doi:10.1097/01.ccm.0000529057.45150.a8

82.   Jevšnik Virant M, Černe D, Petrovec M, Paller T, Toplak I. Genetic Characterisation and Comparison of Three Human Coronaviruses (HKU1, OC43, 229E) from Patients and Bovine Coronavirus (BCoV) from Cattle with Respiratory Disease in Slovenia. *Viruses*. 04 2021;13(4). doi:10.3390/v13040676

83.   Edwards JK, Lessler J. What Now? Epidemiology in the Wake of a Pandemic. *Am J Epidemiol*. 01 2021;190(1):17-20. doi:10.1093/aje/kwaa159

84.   Attanayake AMCH, Perera SSN, Jayasinghe S. Phenomenological Modelling of COVID-19 Epidemics in Sri Lanka, Italy, the United States, and Hebei Province of China. *Comput Math Methods Med*. 2020;2020:6397063. doi:10.1155/2020/6397063

85.   Kin N, Miszczak F, Lin W, Gouilh MA, Vabret A, Consortium E. Genomic Analysis of 15 Human Coronaviruses OC43 (HCoV-OC43s) Circulating in France from 2001 to 2013 Reveals a High Intra-Specific Diversity with New Recombinant Genotypes. *Viruses*. May 2015;7(5):2358-77. doi:10.3390/v7052358

86.   Zobba R, Visco S, Sotgiu F, Pinna Parpaglia ML, Pittau M, Alberti A. Molecular survey of parvovirus, astrovirus, coronavirus, and calicivirus in symptomatic dogs. *Vet Res Commun*. Feb 2021;45(1):31-40. doi:10.1007/s11259-020-09785-w

87.   Jelinek HF, Mousa M, Alefishat E, et al. Evolution, Ecology, and Zoonotic Transmission of Betacoronaviruses: A Review. *Front Vet Sci*. 2021;8:644414. doi:10.3389/fvets.2021.644414

88.   Greenbaum U, Klein K, Martinez F, et al. High Levels of Common Cold Coronavirus Antibodies in Convalescent Plasma Are Associated With Improved Survival in COVID-19 Patients. *Front Immunol.* 2021;12:675679. doi:10.3389/fimmu.2021.675679

89.   Kandeel M, Ibrahim A, Fayez M, Al-Nazawi M. From SARS and MERS CoVs to SARS-CoV-2: Moving toward more biased codon usage in viral structural and nonstructural genes. *J Med Virol.* 06 2020;92(6):660-666. doi:10.1002/jmv.25754

90.   Chan JF, Li KS, To KK, Cheng VC, Chen H, Yuen KY. Is the discovery of the novel human betacoronavirus 2c EMC/2012 (HCoV-EMC) the beginning of another SARS-like pandemic? *J Infect.* Dec 2012;65(6):477-89. doi:10.1016/j.jinf.2012.10.002

91.   Mutiawati E, Syahrul S, Fahriani M, et al. Global prevalence and pathogenesis of headache in COVID-19: A systematic review and meta-analysis. *F1000Res.* 2020;9:1316. doi:10.12688/f1000research.27334.2

92.   Ghandikota S, Sharma M, Jegga AG. Secondary analysis of transcriptomes of SARS-CoV-2 infection models to characterize COVID-19. *Patterns (N Y).* May 2021;2(5):100247. doi:10.1016/j.patter.2021.100247

93.   Viehweger A, Krautwurst S, Lamkiewicz K, et al. Direct RNA nanopore sequencing of full-length coronavirus genomes provides novel insights into structural variants and enables modification analysis. *Genome Res.* 09 2019;29(9):1545-1554. doi:10.1101/gr.247064.118

94.   Li J, Li Z, Cui X, Wu C. Bayesian phylodynamic inference on the temporal evolution and global transmission of SARS-CoV-2. *J Infect.* 08 2020;81(2):318-356. doi:10.1016/j.jinf.2020.04.016

95.   Kiyuka PK, Agoti CN, Munywoki PK, et al. Human Coronavirus NL63 Molecular Epidemiology and Evolutionary Patterns in Rural Coastal Kenya. *J Infect Dis.* 05 2018;217(11):1728-1739. doi:10.1093/infdis/jiy098

96.   Yuan Y, Cao D, Zhang Y, et al. Cryo-EM structures of MERS-CoV and SARS-CoV spike glycoproteins reveal the dynamic receptor binding domains. *Nat Commun.* 04 2017;8:15092. doi:10.1038/ncomms15092

97. Gupta A, Kumar S, Kumar R, et al. COVID-19: Emergence of Infectious Diseases, Nanotechnology Aspects, Challenges, and Future Perspectives. *ChemistrySelect*. Jul 2020;5(25):7521-7533. doi:10.1002/slct.202001709

98. Daniloski Z, Jordan TX, Wessels HH, et al. Identification of Required Host Factors for SARS-CoV-2 Infection in Human Cells. *Cell*. 01 2021;184(1):92-105.e16. doi:10.1016/j.cell.2020.10.030

99. Gautam A, Kaphle K, Shrestha B, Phuyal S. Susceptibility to SARS, MERS, and COVID-19 from animal health perspective. *Open Vet J*. 08 2020;10(2):164-177. doi:10.4314/ovj.v10i2.6

100. Khan MT, Ali S, Khan AS, et al. SARS-CoV-2 Genome from the Khyber Pakhtunkhwa Province of Pakistan. *ACS Omega*. Mar 2021;6(10):6588-6599. doi:10.1021/acsomega.0c05163

101. DeDiego ML, Nieto-Torres JL, Jimenez-Guardeño JM, et al. Coronavirus virulence genes with main focus on SARS-CoV envelope gene. *Virus Res*. Dec 2014;194:124-37. doi:10.1016/j.virusres.2014.07.024

102. Standl F, Jöckel KH, Brune B, Schmidt B, Stang A. Comparing SARS-CoV-2 with SARS-CoV and influenza pandemics. *Lancet Infect Dis*. 04 2021;21(4):e77. doi:10.1016/S1473-3099(20)30648-4

103. Forni D, Cagliani R, Clerici M, Sironi M. Molecular Evolution of Human Coronavirus Genomes. *Trends Microbiol*. 01 2017;25(1):35-48. doi:10.1016/j.tim.2016.09.001

104. Huang X, Dong W, Milewska A, et al. Human Coronavirus HKU1 Spike Protein Uses O-Acetylated Sialic Acid as an Attachment Receptor Determinant and Employs Hemagglutinin-Esterase Protein as a Receptor-Destroying Enzyme. *J Virol*. Jul 2015;89(14):7202-13. doi:10.1128/JVI.00854-15

105. Martínez-Álvarez F, Asencio-Cortés G, Torres JF, et al. Coronavirus Optimization Algorithm: A Bioinspired Metaheuristic Based on the COVID-19 Propagation Model. *Big Data*. 08 2020;8(4):308-322. doi:10.1089/big.2020.0051

106.   Dubé M, Le Coupanec A, Wong AHM, Rini JM, Desforges M, Talbot PJ. Axonal Transport Enables Neuron-to-Neuron Propagation of Human Coronavirus OC43. *J Virol.* 09 2018;92(17). doi:10.1128/JVI.00404-18

107.   Szczepanski A, Owczarek K, Bzowska M, et al. Canine Respiratory Coronavirus, Bovine Coronavirus, and Human Coronavirus OC43: Receptors and Attachment Factors. *Viruses.* 04 2019;11(4). doi:10.3390/v11040328

108.   Kim T, Choi H, Shin TR, et al. Epidemiology and clinical features of common community human coronavirus disease. *J Thorac Dis.* Apr 2021;13(4):2288-2299. doi:10.21037/jtd-20-3190

109.   Sajjad H, Majeed M, Imtiaz S, et al. Origin, Pathogenesis, Diagnosis and Treatment Options for SARS-CoV-2: A Review. *Biologia (Bratisl).* Jun 2021:1-19. doi:10.1007/s11756-021-00792-z

110.   Zhang SF, Tuo JL, Huang XB, et al. Epidemiology characteristics of human coronaviruses in patients with respiratory infection symptoms and phylogenetic analysis of HCoV-OC43 during 2010-2015 in Guangzhou. *PLoS One.* 2018;13(1):e0191789. doi:10.1371/journal.pone.0191789

111.   Morawska L, Cao J. Airborne transmission of SARS-CoV-2: The world should face the reality. *Environ Int.* 06 2020;139:105730. doi:10.1016/j.envint.2020.105730

112.   Zu ZY, Jiang MD, Xu PP, et al. Coronavirus Disease 2019 (COVID-19): A Perspective from China. *Radiology.* 08 2020;296(2):E15-E25. doi:10.1148/radiol.2020200490

113.   Jee Y. WHO International Health Regulations Emergency Committee for the COVID-19 outbreak. *Epidemiol Health.* 2020;42:e2020013. doi:10.4178/epih.e2020013

114.   Shereen MA, Khan S, Kazmi A, Bashir N, Siddique R. COVID-19 infection: Origin, transmission, and characteristics of human coronaviruses. *Journal of advanced research.* 2020;24:91-98. doi: 10.1016/j.jare.2020.03.005.

115.   Briguglio M, Pregliasco FE, Lombardi G, Perazzo P, Banfi G. The Malnutritional Status of the Host as a Virulence Factor for New Coronavirus SARS-CoV-2. *Front Med (Lausanne).* 2020;7:146. doi:10.3389/fmed.2020.00146

Chapter 2 : Immune signatures and predictors of the severity of the disease

Immune Cells Quantitative Abnormalities Associated With Severe COVID-19

Introduction

Coronavirus Infectious Disease 2019 (COVID-19), a disease caused by the SARS-CoV-2 virus (Severe Acute Respiratory Syndrome 2), appeared for the first time in December 2019 in Hubei province in Wuhan (China) in patients who have severe unexplained pneumonia (1). COVID-19 spread to other Chinese regions and then to other countries around the world, which led to it being classified as a pandemic (2).

SARS-CoV-2 virus uses angiotensin-converting enzyme 2 (ACE2) as a receptor, to infect host cells (3). The internalization of ACE2 by SARS-CoV-2 causes disruption of the renin angiotensin aldosterone system (RAAS) resulting in a decrease in the formation of angiotensin 1, and an accumulation of angiotensin 2 with its negative effects (inflammation, fibrosis, coagulation, vasoconstriction). This leads to lesions mainly affecting organs and tissues that strongly express this enzyme, partly explaining the damage to several organs seen during COVID-19 (4). Most people infected with SARS-CoV-2 have mild to moderate respiratory illness and recover without needing special treatment. However, some patients become seriously ill and need medical attention (5). The clinical presentation of this disease varies from asymptomatic forms or mild flu-like symptoms to severe pneumonia with acute respiratory distress and possibly death (6). Old people and those with an underlying medical condition, such as cardiovascular disease, diabetes, chronic respiratory disease, or cancer, are at higher risk of developing the severe form of the disease (7). Indeed, the pathophysiology of COVID-19 is complex involving cytokines storm which leads to inappropriate immune reactions together with enzymes, receptors, and immune cells (8). These immune cells are part of the complete blood count (CBC) routinely requested for COVID-19 patients and therefore constitute a therapeutic follow-up examination of hospitalized patients. Some previous studies have shown that the number of lymphocytes were significantly decreased in COVID-19 patients who needed hospitalization (9). Given that COVID-19 has become an emerging disease, we aimed in this study to determine the quantitative abnormalities of peripheral blood immune cells associated with COVID-19 and establish those associated with the severity of the disease in Togo.

Socio-demographic characteristics of the study population

Male (57.60%) were more represented in the study population than female (42.40%) with a sex ratio M/F=1.36. Most of asymptomatic patients (53.10%) were aged 34 years or less whereas most of symptomatic patients (29.96%) were aged 63 to 92 years. The pupils-student-unemployed group (24.21%) was more affected, followed by artisans-shopkeepers-entrepreneurs (22.30%) and the retired (9.76%). Concerning the comorbidities, hypertension and diabetes were more found in COVID-19 patients with 31.10% and 19.62% respectively, while asthma was found at 3.63%. All symptomatic patients had fever, rhinitis, cough, angina, and angina whereas 92.47% had asthenia and 86.84% had myalgia.

Haemoglobin, white blood cells and platelets count in symptomatic and asymptomatic COVID-19 patients.

Haemoglobin levels were significantly lower (p<0.0001) in symptomatic patients compared to asymptomatic patients. But white blood cells count was significantly high in symptomatic patients compared to asymptomatic patients with a p<0.0001. No significant difference was observed for platelets count (Figure 1).

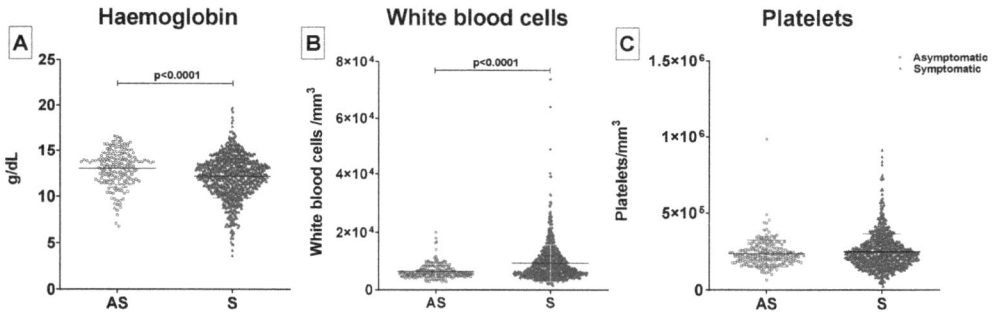

Figure 1: Haemoglobin (A) concentration, white blood cells (C) and platelets (C) count of symptomatic (n=851) and asymptomatic (n=194) COVID-19 patients. The Mann-Whitney U-test was used for comparisons of medians.

Immune cells count in symptomatic and asymptomatic COVID-19 patients

COVID-19 symptomatic patients had significant high count of neutrophils (p<0.0001), lymphocytes (p=0.0047) and eosinophils (p=0.0086) when compared to asymptomatic patients. No significant difference was found for monocytes count between symptomatic and asymptomatic patients (Figure 2).

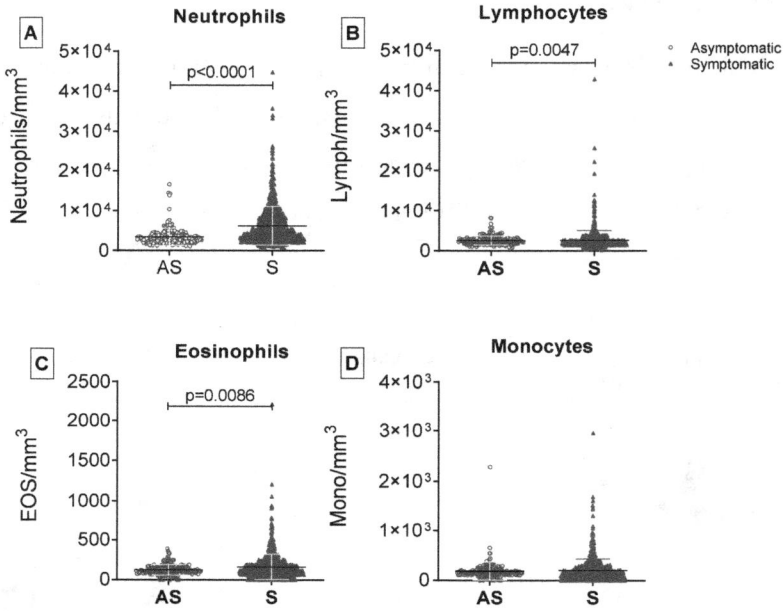

Figure 2: Neutrophils (A), lymphocytes (B), eosinophils (C) and monocytes (D) count in symptomatic (n=851) and asymptomatic (n=194) COVID-19 patients. The Mann-Whitney U-test was used for comparisons of medians.

Contributors to this chapiter

Authors: Gnatoulma Katawa, Christele Nguepou Tchopba, Edlom Pelagie Tchadie, Ayawavi Adeline Hella, Oukoe Marthe Amessoudji, Adjoa Holali Ameyapoh, Essimanam Rosalie Awesso, Awereou Kotosso, Malewe Kolou

References

1.   Zhu N, Zhang D, Wang W, Li X, Yang B, Song J, et al. A Novel Coronavirus from Patients with Pneumonia in China, 2019. NEJM. 2020;382(8):727-33.

2.   Aoun MH, Ben Soussia R, Brahim S, Betbout I, Bouali W, Hadj-Mohamed A, et al. Pandémie COVID-19 : impact psychosocial sur le personnel de santé en Tunisie. L'Encéphale. 2021.

3.   Beyerstedt S, Casaro EB, Rangel É B. COVID-19: angiotensin-converting enzyme 2 (ACE2) expression and tissue susceptibility to SARS-CoV-2 infection. Eur J Clin Microbiol. 2021;40(5):905-19.

4.   Mehrabadi ME, Hemmati R, Tashakor A, Homaei A, Yousefzadeh M, Hemati K, et al. Induced dysregulation of ACE2 by SARS-CoV-2 plays a key role in COVID-19 severity. Biomed Pharmacother. 2021;137:111363.

5.   WHO.   Coronavirus   disease   (COVID-19)   2023   [Available   from: https://www.who.int/health-topics/coronavirus#tab=tab_1.

6.   Cascella M, Rajnik M, Aleem A, Dulebohn SC, Di Napoli R. Features, Evaluation, and Treatment of Coronavirus (COVID-19). In: StatPearls [Internet]. Treasure Island (FL): StatPearls Publishing; 2023. PMID: 32150360.

7.   Sanyaolu A, Okorie C, Marinkovic A, Patidar R, Younis K, Desai P, et al. Comorbidity and its Impact on Patients with COVID-19. SN Compr Clin Med. 2020;2(8):1069-76.

8.   Montazersaheb S, Hosseiniyan Khatibi SM, Hejazi MS, Tarhriz V, Farjami A, Ghasemian Sorbeni F, et al. COVID-19 infection: an overview on cytokine storm and related interventions. Virol J. 2022;19(1):92.

9.   Fathi F, Sami R, Mozafarpoor S, Hafezi H, Motedayyen H, Arefnezhad R, et al. Immune system changes during COVID-19 recovery play key role in determining disease severity. Int J Immunopathol Pharmacol. 2020;34:2058738420966497.

10.   Moueden A. M. BD, Messaoudi R., Seghier F. Profil Hématologique Des Patients Atteints De Covid 19 Au Niveau Du Chu D'oran En Algérie. AJHS. 2021;03(02):22-9.

11.   Wang D, Hu B, Hu C, Zhu F, Liu X, Zhang J, et al. Clinical Characteristics of 138 Hospitalized Patients With 2019 Novel Coronavirus-Infected Pneumonia in Wuhan, China. JAMA. 2020;323(11):1061-9.

12.   Ahmed SB, Dumanski SM. Sex, gender and COVID-19: a call to action. Can J Public Health. 2020;111(6):980-3.

13.   Garcia E, Sanchez-Rodriguez D, Levy S, Claessens M, Van Hauwermeiren C, Taliha M, et al. [Factors associated with intrahospital mortality in older patients with COVID-19 in Belgium : The COVID-AgeBru study]. Rev Med Liege. 2022;77(3):146-52.

14.   Petrilli CM, Jones SA, Yang J, Rajagopalan H, O'Donnell L, Chernyak Y, et al. Factors associated with hospital admission and critical illness among 5279 people with coronavirus disease 2019 in New York City: prospective cohort study. BMJ. 2020;369:m1966.

15.   Huang C, Wang Y, Li X, Ren L, Zhao J, Hu Y, et al. Clinical features of patients infected with 2019 novel coronavirus in Wuhan, China. Lancet. 2020;395(10223):497-506.

16.   Richardson S, Hirsch JS, Narasimhan M, Crawford JM, McGinn T, Davidson KW, et al. Presenting Characteristics, Comorbidities, and Outcomes Among 5700 Patients Hospitalized With COVID-19 in the New York City Area. JAMA. 2020;323(20):2052-9.

17.   Zuin M, Rigatelli G, Zuliani G, Rigatelli A, Mazza A, Roncon L. Arterial hypertension and risk of death in patients with COVID-19 infection: Systematic review and meta-analysis. J Infect. 2020;81(1):e84-e6.

18.   Sayad B, Afshar ZM, Mansouri F, Rahimi Z. Leukocytosis and alteration of hemoglobin level in patients with severe COVID-19: Association of leukocytosis with mortality. Health Sci Rep. 2020;3(4):e194.

19.   Huang G, Kovalic AJ, Graber CJ. Prognostic Value of Leukocytosis and Lymphopenia for Coronavirus Disease Severity. Emerg Infect Dis. 2020;26(8):1839-41.

20.   Shang W, Dong J, Ren Y, Tian M, Li W, Hu J, et al. The value of clinical parameters in predicting the severity of COVID-19. J Med Virol. 2020;92(10):2188-92.

21.   Yang L, Liu S, Liu J, Zhang Z, Wan X, Huang B, et al. COVID-19: immunopathogenesis and Immunotherapeutics. Signal Transduct Target Ther. 2020;5(1):128

22.   Yang X, Yang Q, Wang Y, Wu Y, Xu J, Yu Y, et al. Thrombocytopenia and its association with mortality in patients with COVID-19. JTH. 2020;18(6):1469-72.

23.   Tang N, Li D, Wang X, Sun Z. Abnormal coagulation parameters are associated with poor prognosis in patients with novel coronavirus pneumonia. J Thromb Haemost. 2020;18(4):844-47.

24.   Xu P, Zhou Q, Xu J. Mechanism of thrombocytopenia in COVID-19 patients. Ann. Hematol. 2020;99(6):1205-8.

25.   El Filaly H, Mabrouk M, Atifi F, Guessous F, Akarid K, Merhi Y, et al. Dissecting Platelet's Role in Viral Infection: A Double-Edged Effector of the Immune System. Int J Mol Sci. 2023 Jan 19;24(3):2009.

Chapiter 3 : Hypoalbuminemia, hyper-α-1/–α-2-globulinemia associated to high CRP and IL-6 in COVID-19 patients in Togo

Introduction

COVID-19, caused by "severe acute respiratory syndrome coronavirus 2" (SARS-CoV-2) (1, 2), remains a global health emergency about four years after description of the first case in December 2019 (3). The virus spread worldwide, causing many deaths: as of 5 March 2023, over 759 million confirmed cases and over 6.8 million deaths reported globally (4). In Africa, COVID-19 was not as severe as expected, with regards to the high mortality rate registered all over the world. Over the course of time, molecular biomarkers of SARS-CoV-2 (5, 6) have been identified, allowing the early detection of the virus and also the development of vaccines (7, 8); and consequently, the reduction of the mortality rate (9). As of the time of writing this article, no treatment for COVID-19 is available, SARS-CoV-2 obviously entered our lives and it might be useful to identify other biomarkers to be used for the presumptive diagnosis of the disease.

Indeed, patients with COVID-19 present a large variety of symptoms, ranging from mild such as fever, dry cough, malaise, sore throat, fatigue, pain, loss of taste or smell ; to moderate with dyspnea, diarrhea and pneumonia ; and may progress to severe pneumonia and ultimately to acute respiratory distress syndrome (ARDS), septic shock and/or multi-organ failure (10, 11).

Symptomatic forms of SARS-CoV-2 infection are accompanied by biological changes like increased neutrophil counts, decreased CD4 and CD8 T cells, and in rare cases, decreased hemoglobin and platelets (12, 13). In China, several authors found that an abnormal elevation of the C-reactive protein is observed (14) with immunological disturbances, dominated by considerably elevated serum levels of inflammatory cytokines and chemokines responsible of the so called "cytokine storm". The latter includes elevation of IL-6, TNF-α, IL-1β, IFN-γ, IL-2, IL-8, IL-17, G-CSF, GM-CSF, IP10, MCP1 and MIP1α (also known as CCL3) (15-17) ; and causes tissue damage in the heart, liver, and kidneys, as well as respiratory failure or multi-organ failure (18).

The first case of COVID-19 was confirmed in Togo on 6 March 2020 by WHO (19) and three years later, on 6 March 2023, 808,684 individuals has been tested of which 39,396 confirmed cases, 290 deaths registered and 25 known active cases (20). Data on the inflammatory profile of COVID-19 patients in Togo remains unknowned and the reference method for the certainty diagnostic in the country is RT-PCR. Unfortunately, RT-PCR is not available in most of the hospital diagnosis platforms. Therefore, it appears necessary to find other common biomarkers appropriate and affordable for the diagnosis of COVID-19.

In this study, we demonstrated the implication of biomarkers such as total proteins, C-reactiv protein (CRP), protein fractions (albumin, α-1-, α-2-, β-1-, β-2- and γ-globulins) and pro-inflammatory cytokines (IL-6 and TNF-α) in COVID-19 disease and its severity in patients infected in Togo.

Definition

COVID-19 positive individuals were diagnosed by Real-Time Polymerase Chain Reaction (RT-PCR) in the molecular biology laboratory of INH, detecting 2 molecular markers of SARS-CoV-2 (N gene and ORF1ab) in the sera. They were subdivided in 2 groups by the medical practicians trained for COVID-19 diagnosis following WHO recommandations.

COVID-19 symptomatic: individuals diagnosed positive to SARS-CoV2 and who had COVID-19 related symptoms confirmed by medical practicians following WHO guidelines.

COVID-19 asymptomatic: individuals for who no symptoms was declared or registred following medical consultation. It was about individuals who have been in close contact with symptomatic COVID-19 subjects or have been diagnosed during a screening test for a travel purpose.

Characteristics of the study population

Our study population comprised 74 individuals. Among them, 26 were symptomatic, 18 asymptomatic and 30 negative. The mean age was 46.31 ± 15.60 years, 29.50 ± 8.27 and 29.30 ± 9.70 (p=0.025) respectively for symtomatics, asymptomatics and negatives. Most of COVID-19 positive were male (Table 1).

Elevated total protein in COVID-19 asymptomatic individuals

The profile of total protein shows that there was no difference in total protein concentration between negative and positive COVID-19 patients (figure 1A). However, by splitting positive COVID-19 patients into two groups (asymptomatic and symptomatic patients) and comparing them to negative patients, it was found that asymptomatic patients had a significantly higher level of total protein compared to negative patients (p=0.0302, fig 1B).

Increased α-1 and α-2 globulin concentration and low albumin level in COVID-19 positive patients

The serum profiles of the six fractions of proteins (albumin, α-1/α-2 globulin, β-1/β-2, and γ- globulin) are shown in Figure 2. The analysis of these six fractions revealed that albumin levels in COVID-19 positive patients were significantly lower than those in negative patients (p=0.0001, Fig 2A). In contrast, α-1 globulin (p=0.0005, Fig 2B) and α-2 globulin (p<0.0001, Fig 2C) fractions concentration was significantly higher in positive subjects than in negative patients.

High level of α-1 and α-2 globulin associated with a low level of albumin in symptomatic COVID-19 positive subjects

The concentration of albumin was significantly lower in symptomatic patients than in asymptomatic patients (p=0.0058) and negatives (p<0.0001) (fig 3A). In opposite, the concentrations of α-1 and α-2 globulins were significantly elevated in symptomatics than in asymptomatics and negatives (Fig 3B and 3C).

Symptomatic COVID-19 are characterized by elevated CRP level

A significantly high CRP level was observed in COVID-19 positive compared to negative (p<0.0001). Interestingtly, symptomatic COVID-19 individuals were characterized by elevated CRP proteins and there was no difference between uninfected and asymptomatic individuals (fig 4B).

COVID-19 symptomatic characterized by elevated IL-6 associated to dampened TNF-α

The serum profile of TNF-□ and IL-6 cytokines is presented in Figure 5. Concerning TNF-α, we observed that there was no difference between COVID-19 positive compared to uninfected (fig 5A); this cytokine was dampened in COVID-19 symptomatic individuals compared to asymptomatics (fig 5B). In contrast, COVID-19 infected people were characterized by elevated IL-6 levels; and there was no difference between COVID-19 symptomatic and asymptomatic (Fig 5C and D).

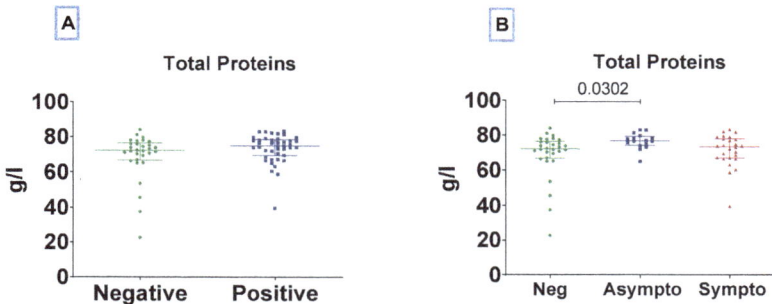

Figure 1: Total proteins profile. Total proteins were measured in serum of subjects. Total proteins concentration data are presented as dot, each representing an individual. Horizontal bars indicate the median with interquartile ranges. (A) The comparison of medians between negative (n= 30) and positive (n= 44) COVID-19 groups was done by Mann-Whitney U test ; and (B) Kruskall-Wallis test followed by Dunn's multiple analysis were performed to compare medians between negative COVID-19 patients (n=30),

asymptomatic (n=18) and symptomatic (n=26) positive patients. p<0.05 is considered significant.

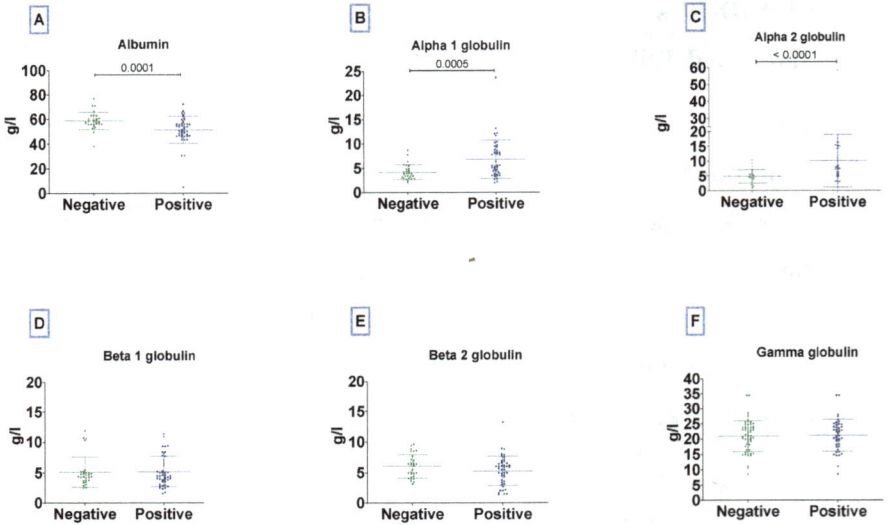

Figure 2: Albumin, α-1/α-2 globulin, β-1/β-2 globulin and gamma globulin profile in COVID-19 infected and uninfected patients. The six protein fractions were quantified in the serum of subjects. Protein concentration data are presented as dot, each representing an individual. Horizontal bars indicate the median with interquartile ranges. The comparison of means between negative (n= 30) and positive (n= 44) COVID-19 groups was done by Mann-Whitney U test. p<0.05 is considered significant.

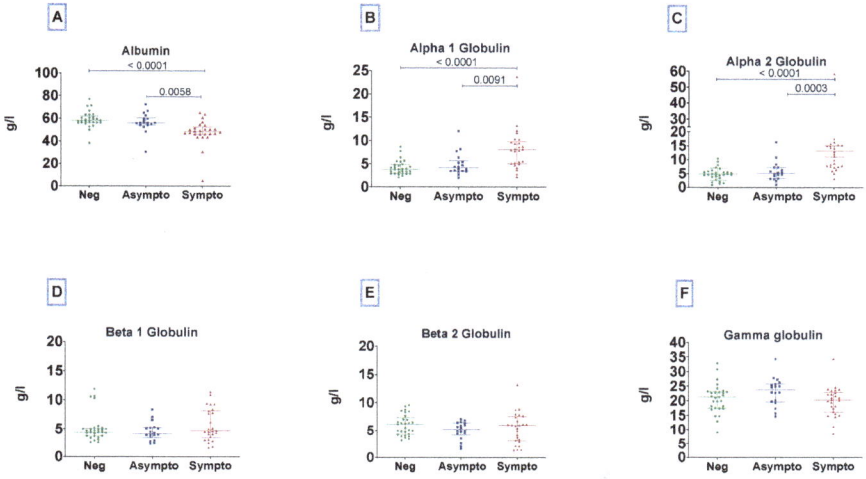

Figure 3: Albumin, α1/α2 globulin, beta1/beta2 globulin and gamma globulin profile in symptomatic COVID-19 positive patients. The six protein fractions were quantified in serum of subjects. Protein concentration data are presented as dot, each representing an individual. Horizontal bars indicate the median with interquartile ranges. Kruskall-Wallis test followed by Dunn's multiple analysis were performed to compare medians between negative COVID-19 patients (n=30), asymptomatic (n=18) and symptomatic (n=26) positive patients. p<0.05 is considered significant.

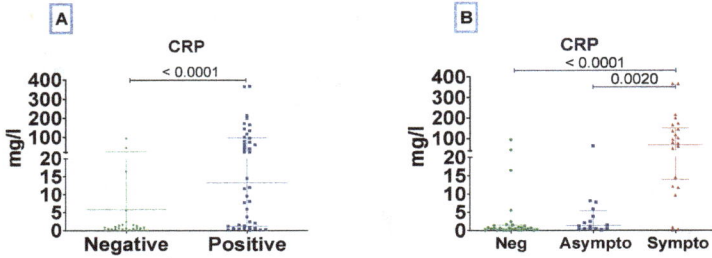

Figure 4: C- reactive protein (CRP) profile. The CRP was measured in serum of subjects. CRP concentration data are presented as dot, each representing an individual. Horizontal bars indicate the median with interquartile ranges. (A) The comparison of means between negative (n= 30) and positive (n= 44) COVID-19 groups was done by Mann-Whitney U test ; and (B) Kruskall-Wallis test followed by Dunn's multiple analysis were performed to compare medians between negative COVID-19 patients (n=30), asymptomatic (n=18) and symptomatic (n=26) positive patients. p<0.05 is considered significant.

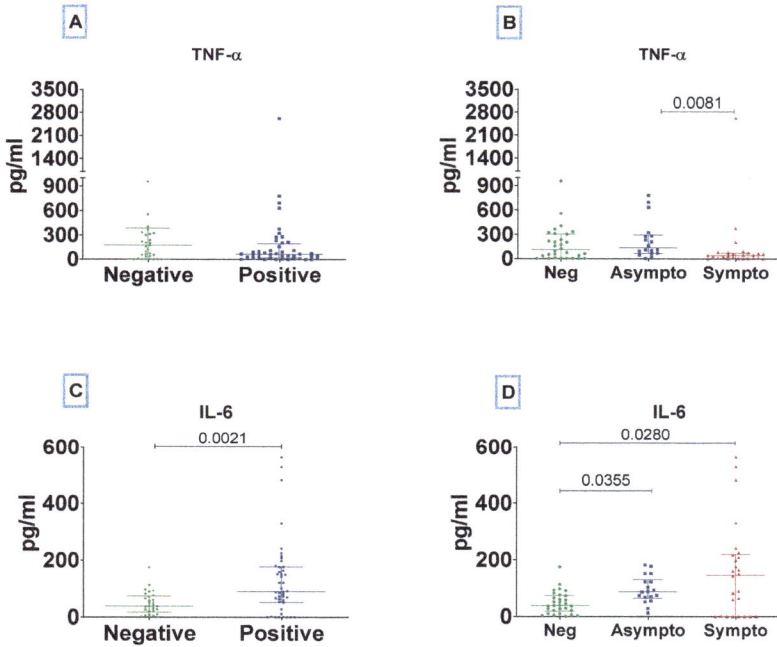

Figure 5: TNF-α and IL-6 cytokine profile. Cytokines were assayed in serum of subjects. Cytokine concentration data are presented as dots, each representing an individual. Horizontal bars indicate the median with interquartile ranges. The comparison of medians between negative (n= 30) and positive (n= 44) COVID-19 groups was done by Mann-Whitney U test (A and C); and Kruskall-Wallis test followed by Dunn's multiple analysis were performed to compare medians between negative COVID-19 patients (n=30), asymptomatic (n=18) and symptomatic (n=26) positive patients (B and D). p<0.05 is considered significant.

Contributors

Christèle Nguepou Tchopba[1], Wemboo Halatoko[2], Yawo Hozo Aloyi[2], Adjoa Holali Ameyapoh[1], Pélagie Edlom Tchadié[1], Marthe Oukoe Amessoudji[1], Simplice Damintoti Karou[1], Manuel Ritter[3], Ameyo M Dorkenoo[4,5], Malewe Kolou[4]

Affiliations:

[1] Unité de Recherche en Immunologie et Immunomodulation (UR2IM)/Laboratoire de Microbiologie et de Contrôle de Qualité des Denrées Alimentaire (LAMICODA), Ecole Supérieure des Techniques Biologiques et Alimentaires, Universite de Lomé, Lomé, Togo

[2] Institut National d'Hygiène, Lomé, Togo

[3] Institute for Medical Microbiology, Immunology and Parasitology (IMMIP), University Hospital Bonn (UKB), Bonn, Germany

[4] Faculté des Sciences de la Santé, Université de Lomé, Lomé, Togo

[5] Division des Laboratoires, Ministère de la Santé, de l'Hygiène Publique et de l'Accès Universel aux Soins, Lomé, Togo,

References

1.   Tchopba C, Ataba E, Katawa G, Gambogou B, Ritter M, Karou S, et al. COVID-19: epidemiology, pathogenesis and immununological basis. Al-Nahrain Journal of Science. 2020(4):1-12.

2.   Al-Qahtani AA. Severe Acute Respiratory Syndrome Coronavirus 2 (SARS-CoV-2): Emergence, history, basic and clinical aspects. Saudi journal of biological sciences. 2020;27(10):2531-8.

3.   WHO. Statement on the fourteenth meeting of the International Health Regulations (2005) Emergency Committee regarding the coronavirus disease (COVID-19) pandemic. . https://wwwwhoint/news/item/30-01-2023-statement-on-the-fourteenth-meeting-of-the-international-health-regulations-(2005)-emergency-committee-regarding-the-coronavirus-disease-(covid-19)-pandemic. 2023;Visited on 10 March 2023.

4.   WHO. Weekly epidemiological update on COVID-19 - 8 March 2023. https://wwwwhoint/publications/m/item/weekly-epidemiological-update-on-covid-19---8-march-2023. 2023;Visited on 10 March 2023.

5.   Safiabadi Tali SH, LeBlanc JJ, Sadiq Z, Oyewunmi OD, Camargo C, Nikpour B, et al. Tools and Techniques for Severe Acute Respiratory Syndrome Coronavirus 2 (SARS-CoV-2)/COVID-19 Detection. Clin Microbiol Rev. 2021;34(3):e00228-20.

6.   Dinnes J, Deeks JJ, Adriano A, Berhane S, Davenport C, Dittrich S, et al. Rapid, point-of-care antigen and molecular-based tests for diagnosis of SARS-CoV-2 infection. The Cochrane database of systematic reviews. 2020;8(8):Cd013705.

7.   Poland GA, Ovsyannikova IG, Crooke SN, Kennedy RB. SARS-CoV-2 Vaccine Development: Current Status. Mayo Clinic proceedings. 2020;95(10):2172-88.

8.   Katawa G, Tchopba CN, Tchadié PE, Simfele CH, Kamassa EH, Amessoudji MO, et al. Systematic Review on COVID-19 Vaccines: Comparative Study of AstraZeneca, Pfizer-BioNTech, Sputnik V, Johnson & Johnson, Moderna and Corona Vac. International Journal of Innovative Research in Medical Science. 2021;6(11):784 - 94.

9.   Huang YZ, Kuan CC. Vaccination to reduce severe COVID-19 and mortality in COVID-19 patients: a systematic review and meta-analysis. European review for medical and pharmacological sciences. 2022;26(5):1770-6.

10.   Alimohamadi Y, Sepandi M, Taghdir M, Hosamirudsari H. Determine the most common clinical symptoms in COVID-19 patients: a systematic review and meta-analysis. Journal of preventive medicine and hygiene. 2020;61(3):E304-e12.

11.   Tay MZ, Poh CM, Rénia L. The trinity of COVID-19: immunity, inflammation and intervention. 2020;20(6):363-74.

12.   Huang C, Wang Y, Li X, Ren L, Zhao J, Hu Y, et al. Clinical features of patients infected with 2019 novel coronavirus in Wuhan, China. Lancet. 2020;395(10223):497-506.

13.   Xu Z, Shi L, Wang Y, Zhang J, Huang L, Zhang C, et al. Pathological findings of COVID-19 associated with acute respiratory distress syndrome. The Lancet Respiratory medicine. 2020;8(4):420-2.

14.   Wu C, Chen X, Cai Y, Xia J, Zhou X, Xu S, et al. Risk Factors Associated With Acute Respiratory Distress Syndrome and Death in Patients With Coronavirus Disease 2019 Pneumonia in Wuhan, China. JAMA internal medicine. 2020;180(7):934-43.

15.   Yi Y, Lagniton PNP, Ye S, Li E, Xu RH. COVID-19: what has been learned and to be learned about the novel coronavirus disease. Int J Biol Sci. 2020;16(10):1753-66.

16.   Liu J, Li S, Liu J, Liang B, Wang X, Wang H, et al. Longitudinal characteristics of lymphocyte responses and cytokine profiles in the peripheral blood of SARS-CoV-2 infected patients. EBioMedicine. 2020;55:102763.

17.   Yang L, Gou J, Gao J, Huang L, Zhu Z, Ji S, et al. Immune characteristics of severe and critical COVID-19 patients. 2020;5(1):179.

18.   Cao X. COVID-19: immunopathology and its implications for therapy. Nat Rev Immunol. 2020;20(5):269-70.

19.   OMS. Epidémie à Coronavirus, COVID-19, le Togo déclare un premier cas confirmé. https://wwwafrowhoint/fr/news/epidemie-coronavirus-covid-19-le-togo-declare-un-premier-cas-confirme. 2020;Visited on 10 March 2023

20.   Gouv.tg. Coronavirus: situation au Togo. https://covid19gouvtg/situation-au-togo/. 2023;Visited on 10 March 2023.

21.   El-Ghitany EM, Hashish MH, Farghaly AG, Omran EA, Osman NA, Fekry MM. Asymptomatic versus symptomatic SARS-CoV-2 infection: a cross-sectional seroprevalence study. Tropical Medicine and Health. 2022;50(1):98.

22.   Neves MT, de Matos LV. COVID-19 and aging: Identifying measures of severity. 2021;9:20503121211027462.

23.   Sohrabi M-R, Amin R, Maher A, Bahadorimonfared A, Janbazi S, Hannani K, et al. Sociodemographic determinants and clinical risk factors associated with COVID-19 severity: a

cross-sectional analysis of over 200,000 patients in Tehran, Iran. BMC Infectious Diseases. 2021;21(1):474.

24.   Farshbafnadi M, Kamali Zonouzi S, Sabahi M, Dolatshahi M, Aarabi MH. Aging & COVID-19 susceptibility, disease severity, and clinical outcomes: The role of entangled risk factors. Experimental gerontology. 2021;154:111507.

25.   Ali AM, Kunugi H. Hypoproteinemia predicts disease severity and mortality in COVID-19: a call for action. Diagnostic Pathology. 2021;16(1):31.

26.   Vavricka SR, Burri E, Beglinger C, Degen L, Manz M. Serum protein electrophoresis: an underused but very useful test. Digestion. 2009;79(4):203-10.

27.   Feketea GM, Vlacha V. The Diagnostic Significance of Usual Biochemical Parameters in Coronavirus Disease 19 (COVID-19): Albumin to Globulin Ratio and CRP to Albumin Ratio. Frontiers in Medicine. 2020;7.

28.   Wang Y, Perlman S. COVID-19: Inflammatory Profile. Annual review of medicine. 2022;73:65-80.

29.   Manjili RH, Zarei M, Habibi M, Manjili MH. COVID-19 as an Acute Inflammatory Disease. The Journal of Immunology. 2020;205(1):12-9.

30.   El Aidaoui K, Haoudar A, Khalis M, Kantri A, Ziati J, El Ghanmi A, et al. Predictors of Severity in Covid-19 Patients in Casablanca, Morocco. Cureus. 2020;12(9):e10716.

31.   Yu C, Lei Q, Li W, Wang X, Li W, Liu W. Epidemiological and clinical characteristics of 1663 hospitalized patients infected with COVID-19 in Wuhan, China: a single-center experience. Journal of infection and public health. 2020;13(9):1202-9.

32.   Zheng Y, Xu H, Yang M, Zeng Y, Chen H, Liu R, et al. Epidemiological characteristics and clinical features of 32 critical and 67 noncritical cases of COVID-19 in Chengdu. Journal of clinical virology : the official publication of the Pan American Society for Clinical Virology. 2020;127:104366.

33.   Peisajovich A, Marnell L, Mold C, Du Clos TW. C-reactive protein at the interface between innate immunity and inflammation. Expert review of clinical immunology. 2008;4(3):379-90.

34.   Sproston NR, Ashworth JJ. Role of C-Reactive Protein at Sites of Inflammation and Infection. Frontiers in immunology. 2018;9.

35.   Han H, Ma Q, Li C, Liu R, Zhao L, Wang W, et al. Profiling serum cytokines in COVID-19 patients reveals IL-6 and IL-10 are disease severity predictors. 2020;9(1):1123-30.

36.   Copaescu A, Smibert O, Gibson A, Phillips EJ, Trubiano JA. The role of IL-6 and other mediators in the cytokine storm associated with SARS-CoV-2 infection. J Allergy Clin Immunol. 2020;146(3):518-34.e1.

37. Frisoni P, Neri M, D'Errico S, Alfieri L, Bonuccelli D, Cingolani M, et al. Cytokine storm and histopathological findings in 60 cases of COVID-19-related death: from viral load research to immunohistochemical quantification of major players IL-1β, IL-6, IL-15 and TNF-α. 2022;18(1):4-19.

38. Shafiek HK, El Lateef HMA, Boraey NF, Nashat M, Abd-Elrehim GAB, Abouzeid H. Cytokine profile in Egyptian children and adolescents with COVID-19 pneumonia: A multicenter study. 2021;56(12):3924-33.

39. Montazersaheb S, Hosseiniyan Khatibi SM, Hejazi MS, Tarhriz V, Farjami A, Ghasemian Sorbeni F, et al. COVID-19 infection: an overview on cytokine storm and related interventions. 2022;19(1):92.

40. Coomes EA, Haghbayan H. Interleukin-6 in Covid-19: A systematic review and meta-analysis. 2020;30(6):1-9.

41. Talwar D, Kumar S. Interleukin 6 and Its Correlation with COVID-19 in Terms of Outcomes in an Intensive Care Unit of a Rural Hospital:A Cross-sectional Study. 2022;26(1):39-42.

42. Tanaka T, Kishimoto T. The biology and medical implications of interleukin-6. Cancer immunology research. 2014;2(4):288-94.

43. Uciechowski P, Dempke WCM. Interleukin-6: A Masterplayer in the Cytokine Network. Oncology. 2020;98(3):131-7.

44. Tharmarajah E, Buazon A, Patel V, Hannah JR, Adas M, Allen VB, et al. IL-6 inhibition in the treatment of COVID-19: A meta-analysis and meta-regression. The Journal of infection. 2021;82(5):178-85.

45. Johnson AS, Polese G, Johnson M, Winlow W. Appropriate Human Serum Albumin Fluid Therapy and the Alleviation of COVID-19 Vulnerabilities: An Explanation of the HSA Lymphatic Nutrient Pump. COVID. 2022;2(10):1379-95.

46. Huang W, Li C, Wang Z, Wang H, Zhou N, Jiang J, et al. Decreased serum albumin level indicates poor prognosis of COVID-19 patients: hepatic injury analysis from 2,623 hospitalized cases. Science China Life sciences. 2020;63(11):1678-87.

47. Scarpa R, Dell'Edera A, Felice C, Buso R, Muscianisi F, Finco Gambier R, et al. Impact of Hypogammaglobulinemia on the Course of COVID-19 in a Non-Intensive Care Setting: A Single-Center Retrospective Cohort Study. Frontiers in immunology. 2022;13:842643.

Contributors

Christèle Nguepou Tchopba[1], Wemboo Halatoko[2], Yawo Hozo Aloyi[2], Adjoa Holali Ameyapoh[1], Pélagie Edlom Tchadié[1], Marthe Oukoe Amessoudji[1], Simplice Damintoti Karou[1], Manuel Ritter[3], Ameyo M Dorkenoo[4,5], Malewe Kolou[4]

Affiliations:

[1] Unité de Recherche en Immunologie et Immunomodulation (UR2IM)/Laboratoire de Microbiologie et de Contrôle de Qualité des Denrées Alimentaire (LAMICODA), Ecole Supérieure des Techniques Biologiques et Alimentaires, Universite de Lomé, Lomé, Togo

[2] Institut National d'Hygiène, Lomé, Togo

[3] Institute for Medical Microbiology, Immunology and Parasitology (IMMIP), University Hospital Bonn (UKB), Bonn, Germany

[4] Faculté des Sciences de la Santé, Université de Lomé, Lomé, Togo

[5] Division des Laboratoires, Ministère de la Santé, de l'Hygiène Publique et de l'Accès Universel aux Soins, Lomé, Togo

Chapiter 4 : Kinetics of cytokines and anti-SARS-CoV-2 Spike Glycoprotein S1 IgM and IgG1 in COVID-19 infected patients in Togo

Introduction

In December 2019, a new coronavirus emerged in China and caused an acute respiratory illness known as coronavirus disease 2019 (COVID-19) (1). The virus was identified as a beta-coronavirus related to the Severe Acute Respiratory Syndrome Coronavirus (SARS-CoV) and was therefore named SARS-CoV-2 (2). In less than two decades, this virus is the third known coronavirus to cross the species barrier and cause severe respiratory infections in humans after SARS-CoV in 2003 and Middle East Severe Acute Respiratory Syndrome Coronavirus (MERS-CoV) in 2012; but with an unprecedented spread compared to the previous two viruses.

Due to the rapid increase in cases and uncontrolled spread worldwide, the World Health Organization declared SARS-CoV-2 a pandemic on March 11, 2020 (3). By then, the virus had infected more than 118,000 people in 113 countries, with 4292 deaths (4). In Togo, the first case was reported on March 6, 2020 and as of November 21, 2022; there were 39323 confirmed cases at COVID-19 with 290 deaths (5).

Although early reports described mainly patients with severe pneumonia (6), the spectrum of the disease is broad, with more than 80% of those infected showing moderate, mild or no symptoms (7).

Early studies involved hospitalized patients with severe or critical illness. In these patients, peak viral load in the upper respiratory tract occurs during the second week after the onset of symptoms, whereas viral clearance is achieved after 10 days in more than 90% of patients with mild disease (8). Elevated cytokine levels, including interleukine 6 (IL-6) and IL-10 levels, increased C-reactive protein (CRP), and T-cell lymphopenia signal worsening disease (9). This inflammatory response disorder is thought to result from an initial alteration in interferon production, which thus reduced early viral control. Early studies in China suggested that anti-SARS-CoV-2 antibody titers are higher in patients with a more severe form of the disease (10). In order to better understand the trends in antibody and cytokine levels, other studies were conducted in patients at different stages of the disease (mild, severe, critical) (11-13).

Knowing that genetic diversity, environment and race may influence the kinetics of antibodies and cytokines while little is known about this aspect in Togo, this study aimed to investigate the dynamics of antibodies immunoglobulin M (IgM) and immunoglobulin G (IgG) and cytokines in COVID-19 infected patients in Togo.

Socio-demographic and clinical characteristics

A total of 80 adults aged between 18 and 76 years were included in the study. The median age of asymptomatic patients was 32 (26-37) years and 56 (46-64) years for symptomatic patients. Most of asymptomatic patients aged between 29 and 41 years old while, symptomatic patients aged between 56 and 76 years old. Male were more reprensted in asymptomatic group and female, in symptomatic group. Regarding the occupation, 60% of asymptomatics were employees whereas 50% of symptomatics were self employed. The togolese in couple were more represented in both group of patients. Principal symptoms recorded in symptomatic patients were cough

72

(60%), fever (57%) and tiredness (48%) and high blood pressure (45%), diabetes (25%) were the most frequent comorbidities found in them (Table I).

Table I : Socio-demographic and clinical characteristics

Variable	Asymptomatic, n = 40	Symptomatic, n= 40	p-value [b]
Median age (Year)	32 (26 - 37)	56 (46 - 64)	**<0.001***
Age groups (Year)			**<0.001***
[18-23[	13 (32.5) [a]	4 (10.0)	
[29-41[	18 (45.0)	3 (7.5)	
[41-56[	8 (20.0)	13 (32.5)	
[56-76[	1 (2.5)	20 (50.0)	
Gender			**<0.001***
Female	4 (10.0)	25 (62.5)	
Male	36 (90.0)	15 (37.5)	
Occupation			**<0.001***
Student	7 (17.5)	1 (2.50)	
Self employed	7 (17.5)	20 (50.0)	
Housewife	1 (2.5)	8 (20.0)	
Retired	1 (2.5)	4 (10.0)	
Employee	24 (60.0)	7 (17.5)	
Nationality			0.13
Togolese	31 (77.5)	36 (90.0)	
Other	9 (22.5)	4 (10.0)	
Marital status			0.11
In couple	21 (52.5)	28 (70.0)	
Not in couple	19 (47.5)	12 (30.0)	
Education level			**0.005***
Not in school	1 (2.5)	5 (12.5)	
Primary	1 (2.5)	9 (22.5)	
Secondary	24 (60.0)	13 (32.5)	
Higher	14 (35.0)	13 (32.5)	
Symptoms			
Fever	13 (32)	23 (57)	**0.025***
Myalgia	0 (0)	4 (10)	
Rhinorhea	6 (15)	4 (10)	
Headache	5 (12)	11 (28)	
Tiredness	10 (25)	19 (48)	**0.036***
Cough	8 (20)	24 (60)	**<0.001***
Comorbidities			
HBP	NA	18 (45)	
Diabetes	NA	10 (25)	
Sinusitis	NA	1 (2.5)	
Obesity	NA	2 (5)	
Asthma	NA	1 (2.5)	
Prostate	NA	1 (2.5)	
Sickle cell disease	NA	2 (5)	
Kidney failure	NA	1 (2.5)	
Blindness	NA	1 (2.5)	

Variable	Asymptomatic, n = 40	Symptomatic, n= 40	p-value [b]
Pleurisy	NA	1 (2.5)	
Hemorrhoid	NA	0 (0)	
HBV	NA	0 (0)	
HIV	NA	0 (0)	

[a] : n (%) ; [b] : Wilcoxon-Mann-Whitney test, Independence chi-square test, Fisher exact test ; * : p-value Significant ; HBP : High Blood Pressure ; HBV : Hepatitis B Virus ; HIV : Human Immunodeficiency Virus

IgM and IgG1 antibodies kinetics

In asymptomatic patients, IgM antibodies raised at D0 were expressed rapidly, peaking at D3 and gradually decreasing until D10. In symptomatic patients, IgM antibodies elevated at D0 were progressively expressed to reach higher levels at D10 (Figure 1A).

In asymptomatic patients, IgG1 antibodies were elevated at D0 and varied very little until D10. In symptomatic patients, IgG1 were progressively expressed and reached higher levels at D10 (Figure 1B).

We observed that IgG1 was less produced in symptomatics compared to asymptomatics at D0 and D3. At D10, IgG1 had quite the same levels in both groups of patients. In addition IgM did not vary among both groups (Figures 1C, 1D).

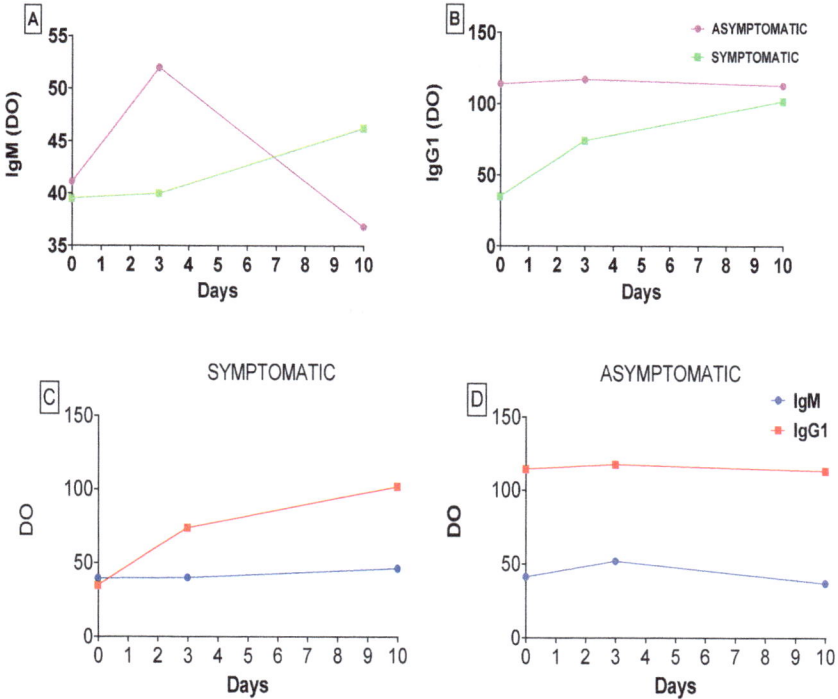

Figure 1 : Kinetics of anti-SARS-CoV-2 antibodies. (A) represents the kinetics of IgM antibodies and (B) IgG antibodies, in the sera of asymptomatic patients in pink (n=20) and symptomatic patients in green (n=20). The mean DO (ELISA) obtained at D0, D3 and D10 was used to establish the antibody kinetics. (C) represents the kinetics of the IgM/IgG1 ratio of symptomatic patients (D) represents the kinetics of the IgM/IgG1 ratio of symptomatic patients.

Kinetics of innate cytokines

IL-1☐ cytokine levels were showed to increase progressively and were similar in both symptomatic and asymptomatic patients (Figure 2A). In contrast TNF☐ levels decreased in both groups rapidly from D0 to D3 and remained constant until D10. However, they were higher in asymptomatic patients than in symptomatic patients at D0 (Figure 2B). Regarding IL-6 cytokine, it's levels were higher in symptomatics than asymptomatics at D0, then we observed a decrease in both groups from D0 to D3 (Figure 2C).

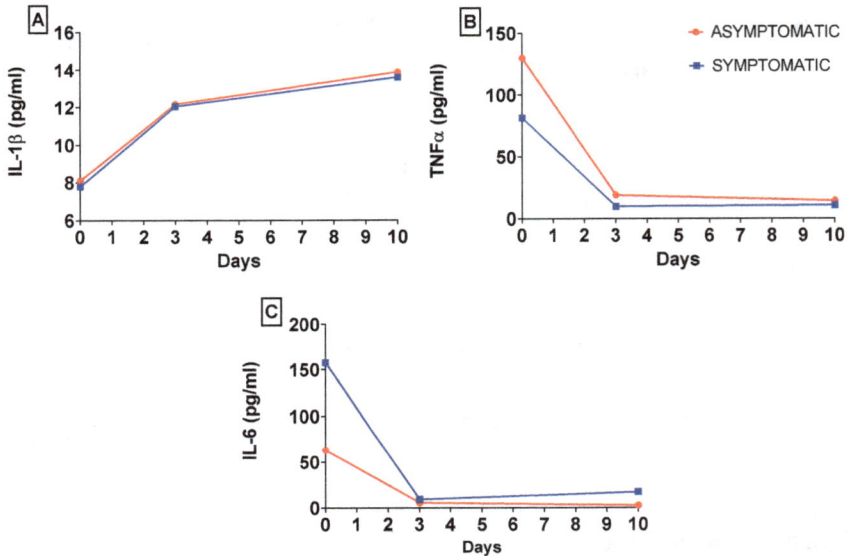

Figure 2 : Kinetics of type I cytokines. (A) represents the kinetics of the innate immunity cytokines IL-1□ (B) ; TNF□ and (C) IL-6 in the sera of asymptomatic patients in red (n=40) and symptomatic patients in blue (n=40). The mean of the concentrations in pg/ml, obtained at D0, D3 and D10 were used to establish the kinetics of the cytokines.

Kinetics of adaptive cytokines

We observed a decrease in IL-5, IL-10 and IFN□ □production from D0 to D3 in both symptomatic and asymptomatic patients (Figures 3A, 3B, 3D). IL-5 was more expressed at D0 in asymptomatic patients and augmented in symptomatic patients from D3 to D10 (Figure 3A). IL-10 levels remained high in symptomatics whereas IL-17A remained elevated in asymptomatics. This latter cytokine increased from D0 to D3 and decreased from D3 to D10 in both groups (Figure 3C).

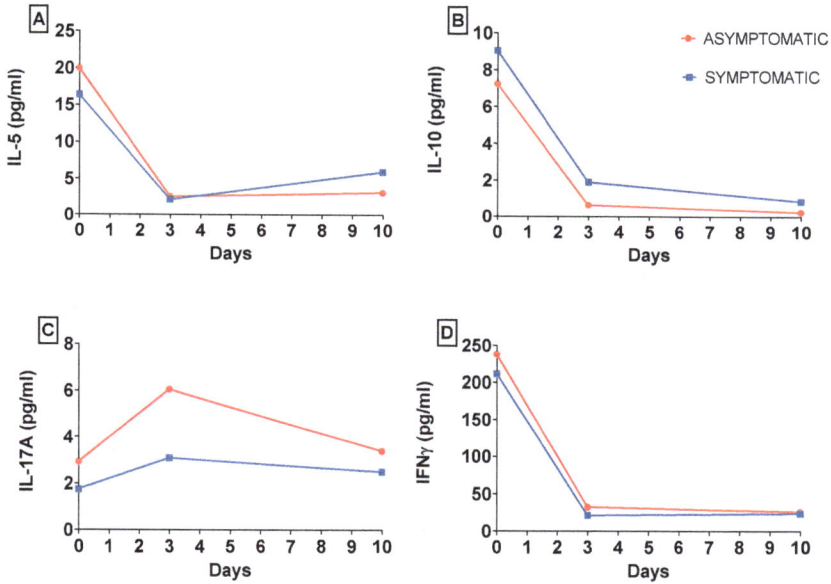

Figure 3 : Type II cytokine kinetics. (A) represents the kinetics of the adaptive immunity cytokines IL-5; (B) IL-10; (C) IL-17A and (D) IFN□, in the sera of asymptomatic patients in red (n=40) and symptomatic patients in blue (n=40). The mean pg/ml concentrations obtained at D0, D3 and D10 were used to establish cytokine kinetics.

Contributors

Edlom P. TCHADIE [1], Wemboo HALATOKO [2], Adjaho K. KOBA[2], Christèle NGUEPOU TCHOPBA[1], Hombamane C. SIMFELE [1,2], Oukoe M. AMESSOUDJI[1], Adjobimey TOMABU[3], Manuel RITTER[3], Ameyo M. DORKENOO[4,5] and Malewe KOLOU [5].

Affiliations:

[1]Unité de Recherche en Immunologie et Immunomodulation (UR2IM)/Laboratoire de Microbiologie et de Contrôle de Qualité des Denrées Alimentaires (LAMICODA)/Ecole Supérieure des Techniques Biologiques et Alimentaires (ESTBA), Université de Lomé, Lomé, Togo

[2]Institut National d'Hygiène, Lomé, Togo

[3]Institute for Medical Microbiology, Immunology and Parasitology (IMMIP), University Hospital Bonn (UKB), Bonn, Germany

[4]Faculté des Sciences de la Santé (FSS), Université de Lomé, Lomé, Togo

[5]Division des Laboratoires, Ministère de la Santé et de l'Hygiène Publique, Lomé, Togo

References

1.   Zhou P, Yang XL, Wang XG, Hu B, Zhang L, Zhang W, et al. A pneumonia outbreak associated with a new coronavirus of probable bat origin. Nature. 2020;579(7798):270-3.

2.   Christèle Tchopba Nguepou EA, Gnatoulma Katawa, Banfitebiyi Gambogou, Manuel Ritter, Simplice D. Karou and Yaovi Ameyapoh. COVID-19: Epidemiology, Pathogenesis and Immununological Basis. Al-Nahrain Journal of Science. 2020:1-12.

3.   WHO. Allocution liminaire du Directeur général de l'OMS lors du point presse sur la COVID-19 - 11 mars 2020 2020. Available from: https://www.who.int/fr/director-general/speeches/detail/who-director-general-s-opening-remarks-at-the-media-briefing-on-covid-19---11-march-2020.

4.   WHO. Coronavirus disease (COVID-19) pandemic 2023. Available from: https://www.who.int/emergencies/diseases/novel-coronavirus-2019?adgroupsurvey={adgroupsurvey}&gclid=Cj0KCQjw2cWgBhDYARIsALggUhrpq7wQ_Z9mekL4MmaDlGau2hVqSI6BPqe_ed5eed0BnG1SFqJk41waAlCPEALw_wcB.

5.   OMS. Epidémie à Coronavirus, COVID-19, le Togo déclare un premier cas confirmé 2020. Available from: https://www.afro.who.int/fr/news/epidemie-coronavirus-covid-19-le-togo-declare-un-premier-cas-confirme.

6.   Zhou F, Yu T, Du R, Fan G, Liu Y, Liu Z, et al. Clinical course and risk factors for mortality of adult inpatients with COVID-19 in Wuhan, China: a retrospective cohort study. Lancet (London, England). 2020;395(10229):1054-62.

7.   Huang C, Wang Y, Li X, Ren L, Zhao J, Hu Y, et al. Clinical features of patients infected with 2019 novel coronavirus in Wuhan, China. Lancet (London, England). 2020;395(10223):497-506.

8.   Vetter P, Vu DL, L'Huillier AG, Schibler M, Kaiser L, Jacquerioz F. Clinical features of covid-19. BMJ (Clinical research ed). 2020;369:m1470.

9.   Han H, Ma Q, Li C, Liu R, Zhao L, Wang W, et al. Profiling serum cytokines in COVID-19 patients reveals IL-6 and IL-10 are disease severity predictors. Emerging microbes & infections. 2020;9(1):1123-30.

10.   Huang C, Huang L, Wang Y, Li X, Ren L, Gu X, et al. 6-month consequences of COVID-19 in patients discharged from hospital: a cohort study. Lancet (London, England). 2021;397(10270):220-32.

11.   Grifoni A, Weiskopf D, Ramirez SI, Mateus J, Dan JM, Moderbacher CR, et al. Targets of T Cell Responses to SARS-CoV-2 Coronavirus in Humans with COVID-19 Disease and Unexposed Individuals. Cell. 2020;181(7):1489-501.e15.

12.   Thevarajan I, Nguyen THO, Koutsakos M, Druce J, Caly L, van de Sandt CE, et al. Breadth of concomitant immune responses prior to patient recovery: a case report of non-severe COVID-19. Nature medicine. 2020;26(4):453-5.

13.   Weiskopf D, Schmitz KS, Raadsen MP, Grifoni A, Okba NMA, Endeman H, et al. Phenotype and kinetics of SARS-CoV-2-specific T cells in COVID-19 patients with acute respiratory distress syndrome. Science immunology. 2020;5(48).

Chapter 5 : Clinical Applications, Future Directions and Predictors of COVID-19 severity

Association between socio-demographic characteristics and severity of COVID-19

Univariate binary logistic regression analysis between socio-demographic characteristics and symptomatic and asymptomatic COVID-19 showed that male gender (OR=1.88; 95% CI [1.35-2.63]); age range [35-47] years (OR=2.54; 95% CI [1.71-3.77]), [48-62] years (OR=5.11; 95% CI [3.26-8.01]) and [63-92] years (OR=21.05; 95% CI [9.98-44.40]) as well as retired patients (OR=24.50; 95% CI [1.51-39.32]) were associated with the severity of COVID-19.

Profession such as managerial and higher intellectual professions (OR=0.162; 95% CI [0.057-0.461]), intermediate professions (OR=0.144; 95% CI [0.051-0.674]), employees (OR=0.215; 95% CI [0.069-0.674]), manual workers (OR=0.157; 95% CI [0.054-0.457]) and Pupils-students-unemployed (OR=0.195; 95% CI [0.062-0.619]) were protective factors against the risk of COVID-19 severity.

Association between comorbidities and the severity of COVID-19

Diabetes [OR = 5.62; 95% CI (3.73-10.78)] and hypertension [OR = 6.34; 95% CI (3.73-10.78)] were associated with the risk of developing the severe form of COVID-19. After adjustment, multivariate binary logistic regression also revealed that diabetes [aOR = 3.61; 95% CI (1.78-7.34)] and hypertension [aOR = 4.76; 95% CI (2.77-8.20)] were indeed high-risk factors for severe outcome of COVID-19.

Association between clinical symptoms and the severity of the COVID-19

Univariate binary regression analysis showed that fever [OR = 36.07; 95% CI (11.62-115.68)], asthenia [OR = 41.30; 95% CI (10.17-167.63)], rhinitis [OR = 10.78; 95% CI (1.48-78.66)], cough [OR = 19.55; 95% CI (8.57-44.59)] and dyspnoea [OR = 9.75; 95% CI (3.06-31.02)] are symptoms associated with COVID-19.

Multivariate binary logistic regression analysis after adjustment showed that fever [aOR = 21.06; 95% CI (6.57-67.49)], asthenia [aOR = 34.17; 95% CI (8.32-140.32)], rhinitis [aOR = 10.17; 95% CI (1.33-32.61)], cough [aOR = 14.06; 95% CI (6.06-32.61)] and dyspnoea [aOR = 6.93; 95% CI (2.09-23.04)] are symptoms truly associated with COVID-19 disease.

Association between quantitative abnormalities of immune cells and the severity of COVID-19

The table 1 shows results of chi-square test and univariate binary logistic regression between immune cells count and symptomatic/asymptomatic COVID-19. The chi-square test showed a link between symptomatic COVID-19 and low/high platelets and lymphocytes count; high eosinophils, white blood cells and neutrophils count with a p value < 0.0001.

From univariate binary logistic regression analysis, it was found that complete blood count abnormalities as low platelets count [OR = 2.75; 95% CI (1.55-4.88)] or high platelets count [OR = 3.12; 95% CI (1.23-7.91)], high white blood cells [OR = 9.87; 95% CI (4.96-19.61)], high neutrophils count [OR = 9.92; 95% CI (4.80-20.45)] and low lymphocytes count [OR = 3.82; 95% CI (2.20-6.65)] were associated with COVID-19 severity.

Table 1: Quantitative abnormalities of immune cells associated with the severity of COVID-19

| Immune cells | Infection status | | X^2 | Univariate analysis | |
	Asymptomatic n (%)	Symptomatic n (%)	p-value	OR	p-value
Platelets			0.000*		
Normal	175 (21.2)	143 (91.1)		1	
Low	14 (8.9)	58 (92.1)		2.75 (1.55–4.88)	0.001*
High	5 (7.9)	650 (78.8)		3.12 (1.23–7.91)	0.016*
WBC			0.000*		
Normal	166 (24.9)	501 (75.1)		1	
Low	19 (18.8)	82 (96.8)		1.43 (0.84–2.43)	1.85
High	9 (3.2)	268 (96.8)		9.87 (4.96–19.61)	0.000*
Neutrophils			0.000*		
Normal	175 (23.9)	556 (76.1)		1	
Low	11 (20.4)	43 (79.6)		1.23 (0.62–2.44)	0.55
High	8 (3.1)	252 (76.1)		9.92 (4.80–20.45)	0.000*
Eosinophils			0.001*		
Normal	194 (19.5)	803 (80.5)		1	
High	0 (0.0)	48 (100)		NA	
Lymphocytes			0.000*		
Normal	167 (22.4)	579 (77.6)		1	
Low	15 (7.0)	199 (93.0)		3.82 (2.20–6.65)	0.000*
High	12 (14.1)	73 (85.9)		1.76 (0.93–3.31)	0.082
Monocytes			0.658		
Normal	193 (18.6)	844 (81.4)		1	
High	1 (12.5)	7 (87.5)		1.60 (0.19–13.08)	0.66

* OR: Odds Ratio; NA: Not Applicable; WBC: White Blood Cells

Inflammatory biomarkers associated with COVID-19 severity

To investigate the inflammatory biomarkers associated to COVID-19, logistic regression analysis were performed. Results showed that IL-6 (OR=1.014; 95% CI [1.005 – 1.024]), CRP (OR=1.034; 95% CI [1.006 -1.062]), α1 globulin (OR =1.518 ; 95% CI [1.165 -1.978]) and α2 globulin (OR=1.378; 95% CI [1.137 -1.671]) were associated with COVID-19 positive; whereas albumin (OR =0.891; 95% CI [0.825 – 0.962]) was associated with absence of disease. After analysis in the multivariate model, only IL-6 (aOR=1.019; 95% CI [1.006 – 1.032]) was related to COVID-19 positive (Table 2).

The relation between inflammatory biomarkers and disease severity is presented in Table 3. In univariate model, the results indicated that CRP (OR=1.063; 95% CI [1.008 – 1.122]), α-1-globulin (OR=1.431; 95% CI [1.093 – 1.873]), and α-2-globulin (OR=1.410; 95% CI [1.128 – 1.763]) are associated with COVID-19 symptomatic status ; whereas albumin (OR =0.878; 95% CI [0.792 – 0.973]) and gamma-globulin protein (OR=0.864; 95% CI [0.748 – 0.998]) were associated with the COVID-19 asymptomatic. Using a backward stepwise logistic regression analysis, it appeared that in a model with CRP, albumin and gamma-globulin protein, albumin (OR =0.713; 95% CI [0.574 -0.886]) and gamma-globulin protein (OR=0.532; 80% CI [0.345 – 0.822]) were associated with the COVID-19 asymptomatic status.

Table 2: Inflammatory biomarkers associated to COVID-19

Biomarkers	COVID-19 (Negative vs Positive)				
	Univarable			Multivariable	
	OR (95% CI)		p-Value	aOR (95% CI)	p-Value
TNF-α	1.000 (0.999 1.001)		0.907		
IL-6	1.014 (1.005 1.024)		**0.003**	1.019 (1.006 1.032)	**0.004**
CRP	1.034 (1.006 1.062)		**0.016**	1.015 (0.989 1.051)	0.409
Total proteins	1.042 (0.991 1.051)		0.107		
Albumin	0.891 (0.825 0.962)		**0.003**	1.009 (0.888 1.147)	0.895
α-1-globulin	1.518 (1.165 1.978)		**0.002**	1.055 (0.713 1.563)	0.788
α-2-globulin	1.378 (1.137 1.671)		**0.001**	1.295 (0.961 2.747)	0.090
β-1-globulin	1.014 (0.836 1.231)		0.887		
β-2-globulin	0.855 (0.685 1.067)		0.165		
γ-globulin	1.012 (0.922-1.111)		0.807		

OR : Odd Ratio;   aOR : adjusted Odd Ratio;   CI : Confidence interval;

Bold values: significant p-values

Table 3: Inflammatory biomarkers associated to severity of COVID-19

| Biomarkers | COVID-19 positive (asymptomatic vs symptomatic) | | | |
| | Univariable | | Multivariable | |
	OR (95%CI)	p-Value	aOR (95% CI)	p-Value
TNF-α	1.000 (0.998 – 1.001)	0.546		
IL-6	1.005 (0.998 – 1.011)	0.142		
CRP	1.063 (1.008 – 1.122)	**0.026**	1.031 (0.982 – 1.084)	0.223
Total proteins	0.886 (0.784 – 1.001)	0.052		
Albumin	0.878 (0.792 – 0.973)	**0.013**	0.784 (0.615 -0.997)	**0.048**
α-1-globulin	1.431 (1.093 – 1.873)	**0.009**		
α-2-globulin	1.410 (1.128 – 1.763)	**0.003**		
β-1-globulin	1.238 (0.936 -1.637)	0.134		
β-2-globulin	1.081 (0.833 – 1.405)	0.557		
γ-globulin	0.864 (0.748 – 0.998)	**0.046**	0.594 (0.375 – 0.944)	**0.027**

OR : Odd Ratio;   aOR : adjusted Odd Ratio;   CI : Confidence interval;

Bold values: significant p-values

Conclusion

We found that low or high platelets count, high white blood cells count, high neutrophils count and low lymphocytes are quantitative abnormalities of immune cells associated with the severity of COVID-19 in Togo. It is therefore important to consider the immune cells profile in the complete blood count examination for the diagnosis and follow-up of COVID-19 patients.

On the one hand, the present study showed that in symptomatic patients, the immune system expressed IgM antibodies first, followed by IgG1 in response to SARS-CoV-2 infection. In contrast, in asymptomatic patients, expression was simultaneous from the onset of infection with higher titers for IgG1. This would explain the non-severity of the disease in some infected subjects. On the other hand, high IL-6 production was noted in symptomatic patients, a pro-inflammatory cytokine that is the predominant inducer of the response in the acute phase of the infection. The present study adds to the theory that IL-6 is a predictor of disease severity in patients with COVID-19. More interestingly, we could observe that the disease is characterized by an upregulation of CRP, IL-6, α-1 and α-2 globulins; and a low level of albumin. Moreover, an elevation of IL-6 level leads to an increase of chance to have COVID-19. These biomarkers may serve as for the presumption diagnosis of COVID-19 disease.